MANAGING DANCE:
Current Issues and Future Strategies

Second Edition

Edited by

Linda Jasper and Jeanette Siddall

Northcote House

To the memory of Peter Brinson
who urged dance to find a voice

First published in 1999 by Northcote House Publishers Ltd,
Horndon House, Horndon, Devon PL19 9NQ, United Kingdom.
Tel: +44 (01822) 810066 Fax: +44 (01822) 810034.

Second edition 2010

British Library Cataloguing-in-Publication Data
A catalogue record for this book is available from the British Library

ISBN 978-0-7463-1203-2

Typeset by PDQ Typesetting, Newcastle-under-Lyme
Printed and bound in the United Kingdom

Contents

Contents

List of Contributors

Deborah Barnard
Deborah Barnard is Director of Ludus Dance Agency and one of four Executive Directors of Dance Northwest. She initially trained in education and specialised in child psychology and dance/movement in schools. In addition to working as an animateur at the Brewery Arts Centre, Kendal, she has been involved in a number of professional committees and advisory boards.

Julia Carruthers
After taking a degree in English Literature, Julia Carruthers worked as secretary to Edinburgh Festival Director John Drummond, and then with David Gothard on the programme at Riverside Studios. She was Programme Co-ordinator at Dance Umbrella before becoming an Arts Council Dance Officer. Now a freelance consultant, her work includes managing the Jonathan Burrows Group and Russell Maliphant.

Rebecca Clear
Rebecca Clear has a degree in economics and was employed as the CCPR's National Promotions Officer from 1996–98. She is now Head of Public Affairs at the CCPR. She is a keen amateur dancer and her interest has included performances at London's Bloomsbury Theatre and key involvement with the Oxford Contemporary Dance School.

Guy Cools
Since 1990 Guy Cools has been working at the Vooruit Arts Centre in Gent. He was responsible for the theatre programme until 1995, and then took over the dance programme. More recently he has curated dance projects in Frankfurt (1997) and Venice (1998). His interest in cultural policy is reflected in his position as Deputy Chairman of the Council for Dance, an advisory board for the Minister of Culture of the Flemish government.

Nikki Crane
Nikki Crane gained her BA in dance at the Laban Centre in 1983 and worked for four years in Scunthorpe as a Dance Animateur before

becoming Dance Officer for Eastern Arts Board. She teaches and performs flamenco and has contributed to programmes on dance and the arts for radio and television.

Sue Hoyle

Sue Hoyle is currently General Manager of The Place. She was previously Education and Community Officer for London Festival Ballet (now English National Ballet); Manager of Extemporary Dance Theatre; Director of Dance for the Arts Council of Great Britain; Deputy Secretary-General of the Arts Council of England; and Head of Arts for the British Council in France.

Linda Jasper

Linda Jasper is currently Director of South East Dance Agency based in Brighton. Before this she was Senior Professional Training Tutor in the Department of Dance Studies, University of Surrey, establishing courses to educate and train students for a range of dance careers. As Dance Development Officer for Berkshire 1982–1990, she created and led a community dance programme throughout the county. Elected Chair of the Foundation for Community Dance 1993–1998.

Sophie Lycouris

Dr Sophie Lycouris is a dance artist and lecturer, currently teaching at Nottingham Trent University. She holds a PhD in the theory and practice of improvisational performance in dance, awarded by the University of Surrey. Her research and choreographic interests include interdisciplinary art practices, hybridity in the arts and connections between movement-based live performance and video-choreography.

Anne Millman

Anne Millman is Director of McCann Matthews Millman Limited, the company specialising in marketing and management for arts, heritage, tourism and voluntary organisations. The company's work covers five key areas: feasibility studies; market research; consultancy; training; and sales promotions. A popular course tutor, Anne's particular specialisms are in market research, cultural diversity and equality of opportunity.

Kari O'Nions

Kari O'Nions is Lottery & Dance Services Manager at Suffolk National Dance Agency. A dance graduate from the University of Surrey, she has also been Community Programme Manager at Suffolk Dance, and editor of the national community dance magazine, *Animated*, published by the Foundation for Community Dance. She has previously written for various dance and arts publications and continues to write freelance.

Sara Reed

Sara Reed lectures in dance studies at the University of Surrey. Formerly she lectured at Chichester Institute of Higher Education. She studied dance at the Laban Centre, London School of Contemporary Dance and Middlesex University, and has taught dance in all sectors of education as well as teaching freelance in the community. In addition to dance education, her areas of interest include dancers' training, health and fitness.

Jeanette Siddall

Jeanette Siddall joined The New Millennium Experience Company in 1998 to work on national education projects. Her career in dance has encompassed dancing, teaching and choreographing, primarily in education and community contexts. She was the first Dance Officer for the South East Region and went on to become Senior Dance Officer for the Arts Council of England. She provides occasional lectures and articles on various dance issues and is currently Vice-Chair of Dance UK.

Christopher Thomson

Since 1991 Christopher Thomson has been Director of Education and Community Programmes at The Place, London's National Dance Agency. From 1986–91 he led the Community Dance Diploma course at The Laban Centre for Movement and Dance, prior to which he worked for ten years with Ludus Dance Company, which he joined as a founder member in 1975.

Foreword

Managing Dance gives voice to the experience of those directly engaged in managing dance. No changes have been made to their contributions in this second edition as their perspectives remain relevant and authentic.

There have been changes in the fortunes of dance since the first edition was published in 1999, and these are summarised by the editors in the following section. In the main, changes have been positive and include the growing popularity and diversity of dance, its raised political profile, new dance spaces and new opportunities for young people. Greater visibility brings its own challenges, and recent years have brought changes in the operations of government policies and departments, and the workings of Arts Council England. These shifts have added new complexities and priorities in managing dance, but its central drive remains constant. Managing dance is essentially about enabling artists to create inspiring work for the largest number of people to experience as audiences and participants. We continue to be in awe of the creativity and effort of all those involved in this process. We thank you and wish you continued success.

Linda Jasper and Jeanette Siddall
2010

Preface

Changes in dance 1999–2010

In 1999 we were on the eve of a new millennium that promised an uncertain but definitely different kind of world. It is a rare privilege to look back and consider the changes that have taken place since then, and particularly to note that the twenty-first century is proving good for dance in Britain. Its growing popularity has been boosted by the iconic film and musical *Billy Elliot* and the astounding international success of the BBC1 *Strictly Come Dancing* series. Audiences for live dance are increasing and new ways of engaging with dance are emerging. The internet carries video clips, art galleries host screen dance installations, television advertisements use dance to promote mobile phones, cars, banking and shoes. Dance in schools and higher education has grown, opportunities for young people to engage and progress in dance are strengthening and diversifying, and site-specific dance productions intrigue the enthusiast and the passer-by.

The popularity of the contemporary visual arts and growing interest in design and architecture are indicators of a more visually literate society. London's successful bid to host the Olympics and Paralympics 2012 is increasing interest in physicality. A more holistic intent towards social policy in health, education and communities, together with a population that is ever more diverse in terms of language, identity and cultural background, all bring dance to the fore as a powerful means of communication, expression and social well-being.

Definitions of dance have shifted. The concern with genre that was evident in the 1990s has been replaced by a fascination with what artists create and communicate. Artists move easily between classical and contemporary genres from across the world. They develop specific and individual movement languages and collaborate with other disciplines to create work for the stage, public spaces and screens. There is greater trust that dance can exist in many forms and locations, and that people can engage with dance in many different ways. The continuum between dance participation and performance is embraced with greater confidence.

The rest of this chapter documents and examines the impact of these and other changes. The section headings used in the rest of the book are used in the same order here, with a couple of alterations. The first of these is the reference to dance houses as these have grown in number and significance since 1999. If we were producing *Managing Dance* today, there would be a whole section on managing dance spaces, but here we are only able to note and comment briefly on their significance. This is followed by dance politics and policies, which is the final section of the book but provides an important context for this new introduction.

Dance houses

Dance houses have been built or redeveloped, creating the beginnings of a building based infrastructure for dance that provides appropriate facilities and brings the benefits of greater visibility, a place to congregate and belong, and homes for an integrated approach to participation, production and presentation.

Sadler's Wells Theatre in London is a particular success story, possibly the only large-scale theatre in the world that presents a full-time dance programme. The redevelopment of the Royal Opera House brought particular benefits for the dancers by providing a sprung stage and studio spaces that removed the need for them to rehearse at the old Royal Ballet School in west London. The Royal Ballet School itself has relocated to purpose-built facilities alongside the Royal Opera House, while Elmhurst School for Dance has relocated to a new building in Birmingham. London Contemporary Dance School at The Place has been redeveloped, and Laban has moved into an architecture award-winning new building in Deptford. Siobhan Davies Dance Company is the first choreographer-led company to build its own home, and like Laban, as part of a south London regeneration area.

A number of national and other dance agencies across the country have converted or built dance houses. These include Derby Dance Centre, converted from a chapel, and Dance City, a new building in Newcastle. DanceXchange in Birmingham is part of a complex that includes The Hippodrome Theatre and Birmingham Royal Ballet. Dance East has built a new home in partnership with developers regenerating the waterfront in Ipswich. Building developments take time. Arts Council England's provision of capital funding through the proceeds of the National Lottery in the late 1990s was critical to making many of these developments possible. Since the withdrawal of this funding route there has been a slow down in the rate of building, sometimes exacerbated by planning difficulties. Rambert Dance is still working towards a new home on London's South Bank, while Northern Ballet Theatre is about to move into a new home it intends to share with Phoenix Dance in Leeds.

Dance politics and policies

In 1999 the relationship between dance and national politics hardly existed. This changed in 2004 when the Parliamentary Select Committee for Culture, Media and Sport held an inquiry into dance development. Select committees cross political parties and have unique power to scrutinise the work of the government and its departments. Usually they inquire into issues and problems. The committee received over seventy written submissions from dancers, choreographers, support organisations and funders which were published alongside its report.[1] Arts Council England commissioned Random Dance to create a short piece to launch the publication of the report, so dance had its moment in the spotlight in parliament. The committee found that dance had achieved much but suffered from a lack of profile and a lack of a building base. Following the inquiry, the government's Department for Culture, Media and Sport initiated a Dance Forum to look at issues that cross different aspects of government. The dance profession is developing its political acumen, with Dance UK focusing on advocacy, publishing the Dance Manifesto with the National Campaign for the Arts, establishing a cross-party Dance Group within parliament and driving DanceVote 2010, a campaign to raise the awareness of dance by parliamentary candidates in the run-up to the general election.

While the promise of the new Labour government in 1997 was realised through significant increases in funding for the arts in its early years, growing pressure on public funds, competing priorities and perhaps a sense of 'job done' resulted in a cash standstill treasury allocation to the arts for 2005–6 to 2007–8 followed by an inflation-related increase for 2008–9 to 2010–11. Rising costs of the Olympic Games had meantime led to a reduction in lottery funds to the arts and other good causes.

Debates led by the new government began with mapping the cultural industries. While this demonstrated the importance of the wider cultural sector, it was also greeted by a sense of disempowerment by those working in the arts who generally felt marginalised within a definition that included industries such as cinema, architecture and fashion. The access versus excellence debate was greatly refreshed by the Secretary of State, Tessa Jowell, publishing a leaflet that posited the notion of access to excellence. This position was taken a stage further by her successor, James Purnell, who delighted the arts world with his defence of excellence. In a speech in July 2007, he stated that: *'...people of every background deserve to have access to the very best, and to have help to become the very best...some barriers are overcome not by lowering them, but by increasing the ability of people to leap them.'*[2] Later in the year he appointed Brian McMasters to lead a review assessing excellence in the arts.

Arts Council England is the major investor in dance as artistic practice. Consequently changes in its structures, priorities and operations have significant impact. In 2003, the eleven organisations that comprised the English arts funding system merged to create a single organisation with nine regional offices and a national office. Regional offices were given delegated powers over funding decisions and relationships with regional partners and regularly funded organisations, providing a single front door for all the artists and organisations based in the region. National office role was co-ordination, national overview and relationships with national partners. New systems were introduced for monitoring investment in regularly funded organisations and a myriad of funding schemes were combined into a single stream called grants for the arts.

The grants for the arts programme distributed lottery funds. It was established without art form budgets and as an open-access rolling programme without deadlines. This brought the benefit of access to larger budgets and the opportunity to apply again if an application was unsuccessful. The move away from art form budgets was disconcerting for artists who were no longer judged in the context of their peers and art form development. Regionalism makes good sense for many public services, but dance is not equally distributed across the country and artists frequently work nationally.

There was a sense of disappointment that the hoped-for benefits of the new single organisation did not fully address regional inequalities and brought new complexities of bureaucracy, particularly in the shift away from art form development, the disjuncture between policy and funding and a more explicit focus on the Arts Council's own ambitions and priorities. A peer review of the Arts Council was followed by a restructure of its national office, shortly followed by the publication of arts policies, a public debate on the value of the arts, a review of shared services across the organisation, a major review of the portfolio of regularly funded organisations and a further restructure that concluded in 2010. While individually, these reviews and changes may have been well-intentioned, it has been hard for those outside the organisation but significantly dependent on its efficient and effective workings, to see the sense or coherence in the whole package.

While Arts Council England had played a major role in the development of dance and its infrastructure in earlier decades, it was the Department for Education and Skills (now Department for Children, Schools and Families), through its Music and Dance Scheme that led the development of pathways for progression for exceptionally talented young dancers. Starting in the 1970s, with the purpose of supporting young dancers and musicians attending one of a small number of residential schools, the scheme expanded throughout the 2000s. It was instrumental in establishing Youth Dance England in 2004 and an evolving national network of centres for advanced training for 11 to 18 year olds, based with dance houses, agencies and professional companies. Separate developments introduced support for students at tertiary level through the Dance and Drama Awards and Higher Education Funding Council conservatoires, and student numbers in higher education have increased by over 50% since 2002–03.[3] The Tony Hall review was published in 2008 and resulted in a new national brief for Youth Dance England to promote opportunities for young people in and beyond school and funding of £5.5 million for 2008/11. This was a welcome and significant investment in dance, but represented only 1.5% of the £363,000,000 invested in similar initiatives in music and 0.7% of the £755,000,000 invested in Physical Education, School Sports and Young People initiative over the same period.

Managing dance artists

A wider range of ways of being a dance artist is gaining recognition and credibility. Choreographers are combining the roles of artistic director of a producing company with work in film, musicals and large-scale site-sensitive projects, and collaborating with the criminal justice system, health practitioners, and scientists. This has always been the case for certain artists, but it is becoming less unusual. It may be a sign of the maturing of the art form that its artists are increasingly curious about and inspired by other contexts and disciplines. Pragmatically, it may be that a mixed economy is healthier and more sustainable, or that new generations of artists are more ambitious for status and material reward. Alternatively, it may be that as the art form grows and finds its way towards a more central role in the life of the nation, that other sectors are more inviting and open to partnerships; that there are more opportunities for dance artists.

Managers still need to believe in the work of the artists they manage, to be skilled at understanding the artist's aspirations and able to translate them for funding or marketing purposes. Even so there are more examples of roles conflating, of artists demonstrating strong business skills and being powerful advocates for their work, and of managers being integral to the process of creative production.

New opportunities for, and a greater emphasis on professional development and leadership have been supported by the Clore Foundation through its Clore Leadership Fellowship Programme and by the Cultural Leadership Programme. Both work across the cultural industries and aim to promote learning across sectors. Dance specific initiatives such as the Dance East's rural retreats for artistic directors of international ballet companies and ballet schools, and the Rayne Fellowships for choreographers aimed to promote connections between dance and the wider world.

The legal and fiscal framework in which managers operate continues to change, and European legislation is a significant part of this picture. The responsibilities of employers emphasise equality of opportunity and the promotion of parental and family friendly working. There has been a focus on governance issues, in part prompted by a growth in the voluntary sector resulting in a tightening of legislation and inspections by the charity commissioners. The spotlight on the responsibilities of running an organisation continues to move, but the intensity of its light rarely dims.

Managing dance products

The spread of the internet has had an impact on the way dance products are marketed. It is almost mandatory for companies and venues to have websites, and usual for tickets to be purchased online. The internet has changed the way we seek and receive information, and sites such as Londondance.com provide a valuable service that would have been difficult to envisage a decade ago. It has also democratised debate about dance with sites such as ballet.co, critical dance and article19 providing platforms for enthusiasts to be critics and give voice to a wider range of perspectives.

Dance made for the screen has also grown since 1999. Channel 4 has been particularly effective in commissioning artistic products that have been innovative and popular. It has broadcast several series of short films, including a series commissioned from Youth Dance England, and commissioned Diverse Productions to work with Birmingham Royal Ballet to create a production of *Romeo and Juliet* with a large group of young people at risk. The resulting *Ballet Hoo!* series of four programmes followed the progress of both young people and artists through to final performance at the Birmingham Hippodrome.

Outside the traditional theatre setting, dance is regularly finding new audiences and creating new relationships with audiences in unusual places. Large-scale productions, such as Akademi's *Escapade* around London's South Bank Centre in 2004, have a massive impact and blur the distinction between artist, audience and participant.

Live touring continues to be of key significance for dance companies. Since 1999 consortia of theatres, Dance Consortium and Dance Touring Partnership, have developed and other signs of a closer relationship between theatres and dance artists and companies have emerged. While positive in many ways, including in developing audiences and encouraging theatres to be more adventurous in their dance programming, it is less obvious that touring for the majority of dance companies has become significantly easier.

Managing dance participation

Ballet Hoo! demonstrated growing ambition among dance companies to make a difference through their education programmes. The role of professional dance in education includes using dance as a means of teaching other subjects, contributing to the dance curriculum, inspiring through performing, creating work and collaborating across art forms. Schools are acquiring new roles in their communities through initiatives such as Academy and Specialist Schools, Extended Schools and Building Schools for the Future, and they are increasingly opening the doors of their dance studios and theatres to the public. The numbers taking dance examinations at GCSE, AS and A level grow and the demand for dance teachers is proving impossible to meet. A new diploma was introduced as part of the reform of the 14–19 curriculum, and dance was one of the pilot subject areas. This growth has been fostered to an extent by greater focus on nurturing creativity, and more so by government targets for young people to engage in physical activity which is creating new opportunities for dance through its collaboration with sport.

The Physical Education, School Sport and Young People (PESSYP) strategy established challenging targets for participation in physical activity through promoting partnerships between activity within and beyond schools. Meeting these targets required an imaginative response to the range of activities on offer, and dance was particularly helpful because of its attraction for girls and those less interested in competitive sport. Youth Dance England, in partnership with the National Dance Teachers Association, took advantage of this opportunity to promote dance. Youth Dance England also established regional dance co-ordinators through project funding from Arts Council England. The ambition was to audit existing provision, co-ordinate and promote activity and develop regional development strategies on which to base a national strategy. This provided a firm foundation for the additional investment that followed the Tony Hall Review and the extension of Youth Dance England's remit.

Youth Dance England was launched in 2004. In addition to the regional and PESSYP projects, provision of information and training, advocacy and conferences, and commissioning dance films in partnership with Channel 4, it has run regular National Youth Dance Festivals. These festivals are the culmination of performances in every region and have prompted a growth in youth dance and the formation of a national performance framework, U.Dance.

Performances created for unusual spaces have become a more visible characteristic of dance, and many include community dancers, students and young people. A film of young people dancing commissioned by East London Dance, *Gold*, was part of the successful Olympics 2012 bid. Dance has been commissioned as part of Open House weekends, and a work for community dancers of all ages has been hugely successful at major events such as British Dance Edition. The distinctions between professional and community dance have continued to blur, and were eroded further by the first Big Dance in July 2006.

Big Dance captured the imaginations of thousands of people. It began as a way of raising the public profile of dance, by positioning it as diverse, fun, for everyone and happening in all kinds of places; initially across London through the Mayor of London's office, then across England through the Arts Council England and the BBC. Over 700 events were registered by groups and individuals on the websites, BBC local radio organised 37 events where 9,000 people took part in *The Big Dance Class*, and the BBC1 programme, *Dancing in the Street* was broadcast live from Trafalgar Square, had a cast of 1,000 and was watched by over 4 million people, a quarter of all viewers of terrestrial channels. It brought together the success of the BBC's *Strictly Come Dancing* and *Strictly Dance Fever* programmes, with the popularity of hip-hop, the drive of world record-breaking attempts to encourage people to take part, and dance as the art sector's desire to work in unusual spaces and engage audiences in new ways. The *Big Dance Class* was choreographed by Luca Silvestrini, artistic director of Protein Dance, who also created *DansAthletic* with 150 young people in and around Canary Wharf station for the launch of Big Dance. Work was created for the sea off Brighton, showing on big screens in Birmingham and performing among the fountains beside London's City Hall. *The Big Dance*, the finale of *Dancing in the Street*, involved 800 dancers and over 40 different dance styles. Big Dance has become a biennial event and the focus of the Legacy Trust regional Olympic and Paralympics cultural project for London and several other regional projects are featuring dance. Managing participation on this scale was a new challenge, but one that is likely to be increasingly in demand.

Some of the issues hinted at in the first edition, such as growing recognition of the contribution that dance can make to health, the development of the role of schools in their communities, and the emergence of dance houses and new dance buildings, and London's successful bid for the Olympics and Paralympics 2012, have added layers of complexity to the relationship between dance as art and dance as participatory activity.

In conclusion

Since the beginning of the new millennium, dance has become more visible in a wider range of roles, settings and contexts. It has grown in popularity and in political importance and is likely that there is a connection between these attributes. As a result, dance artists and managers are managing increasingly complex ways of working. They are subject to new complexities in the legal and fiscal frameworks that affect all organisations and forms of enterprise while moving into less familiar management territory. Such territory includes managing building projects and dance houses, site specific products and more diverse kinds of dance dissemination and participatory projects.

Shifts in the prevailing management culture are placing more emphasis on leadership development, entrepreneurial approaches, partnerships and diversification of activity and income generation. Changes in education and training provision mean that more young people are aiming to enter the dance workplace, but few of them are equipped to work in the areas of shortage. There has been a smaller increase in the number of jobs for dancers than in the demand for teachers, community dance artists, work in health and other social settings, and dance managers but this is not matched in the curriculum of many higher education institutions. At the same time, employers are looking for more assurance of professionalism in the practitioners they employ and models of volunteering and coaching in sport are driving down the expectation of the costs involved. There are not enough practitioners willing or able to move into the emerging management posts.

The state of dance in 2010 seems to be one of growing confidence and new opportunity. At the same time, the difficult economic situation is likely to bring new challenges in terms of funding, demand and changing organisational structures. Dance managers who are equipped to exploit such opportunity and meet new challenges creatively are vital to ensuring the opportunity is not wasted.

Notes

1. House of Commons Culture, Media and Sport Committee, sixth report of session 2003–04, Arts Development: Dance.
2. 'World-class from the grassroots up: Culture in the next ten years.' Speech by Secretary of State, Rt Hon James Purnell MP, at the National Portrait Gallery, 6 July 2007.
3. Burns, Susanne, (2007) *Mapping Dance*, Palatine Higher Education Academy.

Acknowledgements

The staff of the Department of Dance Studies at the University of Surrey for their support and, in particular, Professor Janet Lansdale for making resources available for the production of this publication.

Dr Sherril Dodds for her invaluable assistance and good humour in the editing of this book.

All the contributors who have so generously shared their vision and expertise, and fitted this project into their pressurised work schedules.

INTRODUCTION

Introduction

Linda Jasper and Jeanette Siddall

The business of dance, like that of many other enterprises, depends on creative people. Frequently, the business itself evolves in response to a creative individual's vision, which needs creative people to give it shape, breath and longevity. In dance the visionary is often a choreographer, a creator of dances, but this is not always the case. Creative teachers, dancers, educationalists, policy-makers, animateurs, promoters and managers are equally the heroes of this tale.

This book was inspired by the desire to give voice to the experience of these many heroes, the creative people who daily face the issues and forge the strategies for managing dance. It also responds to the growth of interest in dance and management issues in higher education. Specifically it was prompted by the development of the study of dance management at the University of Surrey. As a new area of study the shape of courses, both at undergraduate and postgraduate level, were directly informed by practitioners and a number of these 'visiting lecturers' have contributed to this book. In consequence, the Department of Dance Studies at the University of Surrey has made a significant investment in its research and development.

Managing Dance: Current Issues and Future Strategies is not just the story of individual businesses; it is concerned with the growth and development of a sector, an art form. Dance has had to struggle for recognition, for the credibility, profile and status that affords it the time and space needed to play its part in the educational, recreational, social, economic, cultural and artistic life of communities. Herein lies a dilemma and a recurring theme of the book. Claiming a place at the table of policy-makers, increasing the profile of the sector, and establishing its role in society (institutionalising the idea) can constrain creativity. Rigid management processes and prescribed expectations may inhibit opportunities for artistic risk-taking. Managers and promoters need to be as creative as the artists in navigating between the institutional and the personal.

Economics is a particular issue for the dance business. It operates in a mixed economy incorporating earned and contributed income, sponsor-ship and, significantly, public funding. A special artistry is needed to translate between the objectives, priorities and accountability needs of the public funding agencies, and the aspirations of choreographers, educa-tionalists and animateurs. It is imperative that the future is artist, rather than funder, led.

Dance occurs in many contexts, and the book draws on a diversity of experience although it cannot cover the entire range of activity. It is organised into sections that focus on the interrelated processes of managing dance artists, products, participation and policies, in order to explore common ground from different perspectives. Many of the issues and challenges are shared, but the most significant unifying factor is the commitment, tenacity and creativity of the people.

1

The Evolution of Dance Management in Britain

Jeanette Siddall

Why does dance need management?

Dance has many manifestations. It occurs in a variety of settings and for a range of purposes, including social, recreational and educational. As a professional art form, dance has to operate in the same political, legal and fiscal environment as any other industry. The majority of performing dance companies are relatively small organisations – few employ more than 20 people and most have an annual turnover of less than half a million pounds. Nevertheless, they must operate within legal structures, observe employment legislation, hold adequate insurance, maintain property and create and sell their products. Creating the product is expensive and intensive, and usually involves commissioning a number of freelance artists to provide the music, set and publicity material. Many independent companies employ dancers on a project basis, and most will have to find and hire the studio space in which the product is created.

Dance companies, the producers, usually cannot sell their product directly to the paying customer. They must work through an intermediary distributor, that is, theatres. The planning cycle of theatres means that the dance company often has to sell the product to the theatre before the product has been created. This then has to be sold on to individual audience members, usually involving further effort by the dance-producing company in collaboration with the theatre. The process of building and developing audiences may involve the company in delivering a range of educational activities in settings beyond the theatre. Any single year may find a dance-producing company creating new work, performing across Britain and overseas, teaching, giving talks, making a film or video or creating work for a specific site or event.

Finance is a further complicating factor. All dance companies are financed through a mixture of public subsidy, grants, and earned and contributed income. Of all the performing arts, dance is the most

5

dependent on public arts funding because it lacks strong commercial, recording or broadcasting sectors. Local authorities support the theatres where dance is performed, as well as National Dance Agencies and community dance, and occasionally provide grants to dance companies. With some notable exceptions local authority grants tend to be small. Sponsors are generally attracted to the larger companies, which are able to provide the back-up and national coverage sponsorship requires; yet a great deal of dance is provided by smaller, project-based companies. Arts funding provides investment for new product and support for touring, but companies still need to market their product and earn income from the box office.

Professional dance is a complex, high-risk industry with a relatively small market. It demands a sophisticated management operation. This chapter looks at the history of the organisational and institutional establishment of dance in Britain and its changing status in British society. The intention is to highlight some recurring themes and points of change that have been significant in the evolution of dance management.

Beginnings of theatre dance in Britain

At the beginning of the twentieth century dance hardly existed as a discreet theatrical activity. While a few theatres had their own ballet companies, such as the Empire Theatre in London which had hosted a resident ballet company since 1887 and included Adeline Genée, Lydia Kyasht and Phyllis Bedells among its ballerinas, the ballets they presented formed part of a mixed programme. Their titles suggest a degree of topicality, such as *Paris Exhibition*, and a concern with situations or activities familiar to a popular audience, for example *The Sports of England, By the Sea* or *The Press*. As a diversion within a mixed programme, dance did not have to run its own organisations or attract a specialist audience.

Music Hall attracted a popular audience, providing a welcome distraction from a hard, often cruel life for a population that was largely illiterate and whose homes offered few comforts. During the 1840s and 1850s a number of theatres were built that were capable of seating large audiences. For example, the East London Theatre in Stepney held 2150, the Standard in Shoreditch 3400, and the Britannia in Hoxton 5000. All were within a few miles of each other (Pick, 1983). In the 1860s the Bancrofts, the Haymarket Theatre managers, introduced mechanisms designed to deter the masses in favour of a more refined audience. These included carpeting and decoration, raising admission prices and doing away with the custom of reducing prices after nine o'clock. Single plays, generally reflecting the interests and morals of the middle classes, were presented. Theatres built in London between 1865 and 1885 had smaller seating capacities, none more than 1500 and several about 650. Smaller theatres were more intimate, suited to straight plays rather than spectacle, and had a greater appeal for the middle classes. They also required higher seat prices in order to maintain a profit. In 1879 admission prices in London ranged between six pence and two shillings for the large music halls and between two shillings and ten shillings and six pence for the more fashionable theatres. By the turn of the century theatre had diversified to suit and reflect the tastes and habits of different social classes.

This period saw the establishment of a new distinction between 'art' and 'entertainment', in which the former was elevated and the latter denigrated. Dance was firmly identified with the latter. In part this resulted from the association between the activity and the places in which it occurred, namely the music halls. Victorian attitudes to the body and the strict moral codes of the period also contributed to the low status accorded to dance. During Elizabethan times the ideals of the Renaissance had sought balance between the physical spiritual and intellectual. By Victorian times the intellectual and spiritual had gained dominance while the physical was deemed primitive or immoral. The Public Health Act of 1890 required all premises, including those already licensed for the selling and consuming of liquor, to be licensed by the local authority before they could be used for singing or dancing. The Act was still in force in many parts of the country in the 1980s (Arnold-Baker, 1983).

With no organisational base, limited performance opportunities, low status and little in the way of professional support, it is hardly surprising that dance had a low profile in Britain at the beginning of the twentieth century. It was, however, starting to make an impact in education, essentially as a form of physical training for girls. Middle-class girls studied dance as a means of improving their deportment, grace and musicality. In addition there were a number of experiments in developing dance as an expressive form. But it was not until the arrival of Diaghilev's Ballets Russes that one form of dance, ballet, attained the respectability that was the prerequisite for its establishment as an art form in its own right.

Transplanting respectable roots

Diaghilev's 1909 Paris season was intended to focus on opera. It was to have been presented under the patronage of the Grand Duke Vladimir, which would have guaranteed Imperial subsidy, but an accident of history opened a chink in the barricade of respectability. The sudden death of Vladimir resulted in the loss of any hope of subsidy and, in an attempt to reduce the costs of the season, a greater proportion of ballet was included as it was cheaper to produce than opera. The change in programme required a new venue because the Paris Opera was deemed too superior to host a whole evening of ballet. According to the theatre's management:

> [because of] the unique position of the Opera as one of the French National Theatres, it could not possibly be let for mere ballet performances. Ballet is not art of the kind that could possibly be shown by itself at the Opera within whose precincts there was no place for such a thing.
>
> Grigorovich (1953, p.14)

Finding an alternative suitable venue was no easier in Paris in 1909 than it is in London today. The Théâtre du Châtelet was chosen (it was smaller and far more modest than the Opera), but Diaghilev's efforts in refurbishing the theatre and winning the support of influential journalists, socialites and artists contributed significantly to the season's critical and financial success.

Money was a constant worry throughout the 20 years of Ballet Russes existence. The early London seasons were sponsored by Sir Joseph Beecham, but World War I put an end to this arrangement. The 1918/19 season was spent entirely in London, where the company gave 12 performances a week of short ballets as part of the music hall programmes at the Coliseum, followed by a three-month season of full-length ballets at the Alhambra. In 1922, Sir Oswald Stoll financed the evening-length production of *The Sleeping Princess* in the expectation that – much as musicals are today – a long-running production would be more financially viable than a short season of many different ballets. Unfortunately this proved not to be the case. The audience for ballet was not sufficiently large to sustain a long run, and *The Sleeping Princess* was forced to close prematurely. Consequently, the Company was unable to perform in England for four years, and it took three seasons at the Coliseum before the debts were paid off. Diaghilev was in debt to Stoll who sequestered the sets and costumes. The dancers also suffered financial worries, and in 1925 they threatened to strike unless they received a pay increase.

The Ballet Russes roamed the major cities of Europe and North and South America in an effort to find new audiences. By contemporary standards its seasons were long. Its audience was predominantly drawn from the wealthy and fashionable who were attracted by the company's reputation, its collaboration with the more established arts of music and painting, and by its spectacle and exclusivity. Grigoriev, Diaghilev's repetiteur, described the audience at the opening of the 1928 London season:

In those days the stalls and boxes in London would still be filled by ladies in evening gowns and men in tail-coats; and the sight of such elegance was always a stimulus to the dancers. The company in any case loved performing in London. They found the audiences much more responsive than in Paris; and individuals were flattered at being singled out. In Paris attention was fixed almost exclusively on composers, designers and choreographers, the performers, with rare exceptions, being relegated to the background.

Grigoriev in Grigorovich (1953, p.247)

British regional audiences were less receptive. Grigoriev describes the 1920 tour tersely:

The public we confronted showed little interest in ballet and found our performances merely bewildering... our financial position was hardly improved by our agent in Birmingham, who made off with the takings.

Grigoriev in Grigorovich (1953, p.158)

A number of themes familiar to contemporary managers of dance can be detected in the story of the Ballets Russes: low status, poor pay for dancers, the difficulty of finding appropriate venues, continual touring, and the need to build audiences. The rich, influential and respectable audiences who attended the Ballet Russes performances were essential to the establishment of English Ballet.

Institutionalisation

The Imperial Russian Ballet that made Diaghilev's enterprises possible was supported, indeed owned, by the Russian Court. It was firmly patriarchal and the dancers were members of the royal household. Diaghilev operated a more liberal brand of patronage, dependent on a few, very wealthy individuals who were prepared to initiate activity that would then be available to many at less than the actual cost. When it worked well the few benefited financially, but their prime motivation was their belief in Diaghilev's vision. There was no need for them to act collectively, or to consider the long-term impact of their actions. With the death of Diaghilev came the demise of his company. If ballet was to take root in England it needed an organisational base that went beyond a single vision dependent on patronage.

The institutionalisation of culture is a recognised phenomenon. As Paul DiMaggio suggests in his description of the creation of an organisational base for high culture in America: 'In almost every literate society, dominant status groups or classes eventually have developed their own styles of art and the institutional means of supporting them' (1991). The extent to which ballet was inherently such an art, or whether the supporters of the art choose to ally themselves to the appropriately dominant groups as a means of securing institutional support, is arguable. Events are rarely so polarised, or so planned. That institutionalisation occurred and was an imperative is certain. The process includes establishing organisations, and goes beyond the tangible, visible entities of organisations. It encompasses notions of acceptance, recognition, status and power, and the outcome of the process of institutionalisation is to endow the subject with these qualities. Setting rules that define the chosen subject, and exclude other lesser activities, is an effective means of promoting this process.

England had begun to set rules for the teaching of ballet around the turn of the century. In 1920 the Dancers' Circle was formed, bringing together teachers of various dance styles to agree a standard syllabus and establish examinations. This initiative proved hugely successful, with 161 candidates examined in the first year. Higher level examinations were introduced together with grade examinations for children. By 1926 there were over 800 members and by 1928 over 2000 children were entered for each grade examination. The organisation became the Royal Academy of Dancing, which today is a significant multi-national industry, holding examinations in over 60 countries throughout the world.

The development of committees, planning and expansionist strategies were key to the establishment of the organisational base for dance in England in the twentieth century. The Dancers' Circle had been instigated by Philip Richardson, who almost ten years later founded another committee, the Camargo Society, to provide performance opportunities for the fledgling English ballet. In many ways the model was not dissimilar to the showcases mounted by 'independent' dancers in the 1970s. Both were produced by committee, overtly democratic and self-financing with the consequent low budgets and attendant financial crises. (Where the two differed was in the social class of the protagonists.) The Camargo Society enabled the creation of a number of ballets, which were eventually given over to Ninette de Valois's Vic-Wells Ballet.

De Valois and Marie Rambert, both of whom had danced with Diaghilev, had visions for an English ballet. Both opened schools in the 1920s and mounted performances of their students. It appears, however, that there was only room for one national ballet, a cause championed by Arnold Haskell in his book *The National Ballet* published in 1943. His criteria for a national ballet conveniently described the characteristics of the Sadler's Wells Ballet (as the Vic-Wells Ballet had become):

A fixed domicile, school attached to the theatre and the majority of the dancers and the staff belonging to the country of domicile...a permanent repertoire of 'museum' pieces that are the classical foundations of the art.

Haskell (1944, p.32)

The desire was less for a national institution that would provide an organisational base for an indigenous art form, more for an imported art form to be accepted as a responsibility of the nation. Eventually the work of English choreographers would be added to the repertoire of 'museum' pieces, but the language and conventions remained essentially of foreign extract.

Sadler's Wells Ballet did become the national ballet, The Royal Ballet, consisting of a resident company, a touring company and a school. This was not as a result of a national policy, as noted by A.V. Coton writing in 1961:

I do not think I ask too much in wanting – as I wanted at the time – all our ability, ideas, talents, to be utilised for the glory and advancement of the idea of English Ballet. But Fate – which is another name for pressure groups, prestige seekers, propagandists – willed otherwise. The Sadler's Wells company became by a stroke of the pen, not by artistic leadership, the English National Ballet.

Coton (1975, p.44)

During the 1930s a number of companies were set up. The number actually grew during, and perhaps because of, World War II. All were self-financing. The most fortunate had rich patrons, but many eked out a precarious existence, frequently dependent on the goodwill of the dancers. Ballet had become a popular art form.

Ballet and the beginnings of public subsidy

World War II had a dramatic effect on the civilian population. Established social structures were dismantled as fathers and sons were conscripted, children evacuated, women went to work, and bombing and rationing disrupted the lives of everyone. This dismantling caused some concern among a number of like-minded individuals who saw a civilising value in the arts in their capacity to promote social cohesion and individual inspiration. The Council for the Encouragement of Music and the Arts (CEMA) was set up, with funding from the American Pilgrim Trust matched by funds from the Government, to encourage the making of music and plays by the populace. An incidental objective was to provide support for professional singers and players who 'may suffer from a lack of demand for their work'.

Government had already given financial assistance for artistic activity through museums and galleries, the BBC, the British Film Institute and military bands. In 1930, the government had provided £40000 to Covent Garden Opera through the BBC (Jenkins, 1979). CEMA was different in that it was a conspicuous agency of State support and not only concerned with giving aid to buildings or established institutions. Initially CEMA promoted amateur work and gave out small grants. It was established and run by a committee, later called the Council, and it was rooted in notions of education, participation and public benefit. Its instigators included William Emrys Williams (secretary of the British Institute of Adult Education), Walford Davies, and Ralph Vaughan Williams. A change of direction occurred when John Maynard Keynes became chairman in 1942. Lord Clark, director of the National Gallery, described him as: 'not the man for wandering minstrels and amateur theatricals. He believed in excellence' (Baldry, 1981). Although established as a temporary mechanism to deal with the particular circumstances of a country at war, CEMA was to become, with hardly any changes, the Arts Council of Great Britain. With the rise of the Arts Council, it has been argued, state patronage replaced private patronage.

At the beginning of the war, the Entertainment National Service Association (ENSA) provided the route for government funding of ballet. ENSA was funded through the armed services vote and was run by Basil Dean. As its name suggests, it was concerned with providing entertainment for the armed services and it counted the Sadler's Wells Ballet among such entertainment. CEMA, on the other hand, ignored ballet until 1942 when Keynes's concern for excellence and personal interest in ballet (he was married to former Diaghilev dancer Lydia Lopokova) was instrumental in introducing tours by dance companies. In 1943 CEMA brought together the disbanded Ballets Jooss and toured the Sadler's Wells Ballet, announcing this new departure in its *March Bulletin*:

> CEMA began by ruling out ballet and opera. This was done arbitrarily and of set purpose, in order that the first programmes might be shaped with definite limits and with some degree of concentration. The limits are, very properly, expanding and already three ballet companies are at work. The third is Rambert, which has also been gathered together again and is going out on a tour of the hostels on March 29th. It will be the first to take ballet to the munitions workers, and we hope its members will find their new audiences as satisfying as our actors and musicians have done.
>
> CEMA (1943)

Given that there is little evidence of such purpose in 1939, the accuracy of this statement might be questioned. It may be, however, that the change in CEMA's attitude to ballet indicates a shift in the status of the art form. Its popularity in the 1930s had made it an appropriate activity for ENSA, but not sufficiently worthy for the educational purposes of CEMA. Keynes's concern with the professional arts and his particular interest in ballet provided an opportunity to raise its status from entertainment to art, and to bring it into the fold of public subsidy. The February 1942 bulletin had made significant claims for 'the worthiness of the CEMA audience':

> We believe the CEMA audiences are not of the kind to be deterred by a rough or icy evening; indeed we have abundant evidence of long journeys made at the end of a long day's work to enjoy good music or plays.
>
> CEMA (1942)

The extent to which the CEMA audience could be distinguished from the audiences who supported ENSA's activities, or those who flocked to the cinema or the dance-halls, was spurious. The demarcation between art and entertainment was being strengthened and extended to the audience. This may have been useful in justifying special treatment for certain activities, but it also gave rise to subsequent concerns with audience development, marketing and education in, rather than through, the arts.

CEMA also established touring patterns for dance companies. The Sadler's Wells Ballet spent the most time in London and other major cities; Ballets Jooss toured more widely; Ballet Rambert toured most extensively to a wide range of smaller venues, often for single performances. The large-, middle- and small-scale approach to national touring that can be detected in CEMA's tours remains pertinent today, even though there are more companies and the picture is more complex.

Dealing with diversity

The 1950s and 1960s saw the development of what the American economist J.K Galbraith termed 'the affluent society'. In 1951 there were 2.5 million private cars and one million television sets in Britain; by 1964 there were 8 million cars and 13 million television sets. There was an increase in the number of households owning refrigerators and telephones and in people taking holidays abroad (May, 1987). The dramatic increase in the standard of living was reflected in an expansiveness in education, legislation and social reform. The death penalty was abolished in 1965, homosexual acts between consulting adult males were legalised in 1967, new universities were founded, and the Open University was established in 1969.

Jennie Lee, Minister for the Arts, published a white paper *A Policy for the Arts – The First Steps* in 1965. As the first government white paper to concentrate on the arts, it firmly established arts provision as a concern of government. Private patronage, however, was, once again, to have the most significant impact on dance. Martha Graham brought her pioneering modern dance company to London for the first time in March 1954. This was a very different form of dance to anything that had been seen previously in Great Britain. From America, London was seen as the artistic centre of Europe and consequently the most important place to succeed. Despite the fact that they often performed for no more than one night in New York, the company gave a two-week season in London. It was not a success. As Robert Cohan, a dancer with the company at the time, recalled:

> We were totally devastated to be completely rejected here – but completely. Almost all the critics, one after another, said that this was an absurd way to move, an absurd idea of dance, there was no technique to start with, it was boring, it was ugly, it was stupid – one review after another. There was one night when there were only thirty people in the audience.
>
> White (1985, p.114)

Robin Howard was among those small audiences, and his enthusiasm and generosity persuaded the company to return to Britain in 1963, when he backed seasons in London and Edinburgh. Happily, the performances in Edinburgh were such a success that by the time the company reached London the season was almost sold out. Such was the interest from the dance world, notably from Marie Rambert, that Howard established a trust fund to enable British dancers to train with Graham in America. In 1964 there was something of an invasion of American contemporary dance, with the companies of Merce Cunningham, Alvin Ailey and Paul Taylor providing a total of 13 weeks of performances. In 1965, ballet dancers and dancers from Graham's company shared the same stage in a programme given by the Royal Ballet's *Ballet for All* under the direction of Peter Brinson. Regular classes were set up and grew into a school by the following year.

The Contemporary Ballet Trust was formed in July 1966; the word 'ballet' being more respectable than 'dance', which at that time was too closely connected to dance halls. Just as Diaghilev's collaboration with leading artists from established, respectable disciplines had legitimised ballet, the term 'ballet' now legitimised a dance form whose aesthetic principles were very different. The patrons of the new trust were drawn from a range of artistic disciplines: Henry Moore, Lord Harewood, John Gielgud, Marie Rambert, Dame Ninette de Valois and Martha Graham. Gradually the school developed a full-time three-year course and gave birth to a company, whose early performances were supplemented by dancers from the Graham Company. Robert Cohan was appointed artistic director in 1967, and in 1969 the Trust took over The Place to provide a home for the school, the company and The Place Theatre. American contemporary dance had established English roots.

A range of other developments took place during the 1960s. In 1966 Marie Rambert restructured her company into an ensemble to perform contemporary work under the directorship of Norman Morrice. It took four months to reorganise and rehearse the company, made financially possible because the company was funded by the Arts Council, and had been since the days of CEMA. The Arts Council was able to respond to change by an established organisation, but responding to the myriad of experiment promulgated by the pioneers of New Dance was more difficult. As 'a revolution which has partly been about choreographic experiment and partly about altering the way people think about dance' (Mackrell 1992, p.1), New Dance challenged not only the content of the form but the way in which it was organised and presented. It challenged accepted conventions about what constituted performance and theatricality, the relationship between choreographer and dancer, and between performer and audience. It took place in unusual spaces, at unusual times and embraced all forms of dance as being as equally valid and legitimate. It sought to remove the barriers that isolated dance from the real world and to gain recognition for dance as part of living. It was the beginning of a more explicit politicisation of dance.

It would be naive to suggest that dance had been apolitical up to this point. Establishing institutions, gaining acceptance and status as 'art', and achieving a place at the public subsidy table had all been political acts, won through recognising and exploiting contemporary political imperatives. One of the differences between the 1960s and 1970s was that in the 70s it was British dancers seeking their own voice and validity for their own experiment, rather than individual entrepreneurs working to import an established entity. In the past it was the political environment that was different, with art as much an aspect of government as health or education, although with a lower status as indicated by the lack of a seat in the inner cabinet of government. The existence of the Arts Council was, however, tangible proof of government commitment to funding the arts, although in 1960 about one-third of the total Arts Council grant went to the Royal Opera House and just over two per cent went to the rest of dance, mostly to ballet.

Dance was administered through the music department. There was no separate dance department until 1979, by which time the total Arts Council grant had grown from £1.5 million to £63 million, with 11 per cent going to the Royal Opera House and just over 3 per cent to the rest of dance. The Arts Council had operated an unashamed hierarchy of art forms since the days when CEMA had selected music and drama as the forms most appropriate to its initial objectives. That dance took second place to music was signalled by the fact that, although the ballet was resident first and had two companies, the jewel in the national arts crown was named the Royal Opera House, never the Royal Ballet House. This understanding was made explicit by Eric W. White, assistant secretary to the Arts Council from 1942 to 1971:

> If composers are mentioned first when one discusses the ballet 'classics' to be included in the current repertory of an international company like the Royal Ballet, this is because music has priority over movement – it provides the time framework within which the dance creation takes place.
>
> White (1975)

In 1966 an opera and ballet enquiry was set up, with a separate sub-committee for ballet. As a result, London Contemporary Dance Theatre was 'adopted' by ballet and a new fund was formed to 'assist creativity in ballet and in the new forms of dance theatre which are evolving from it'. This suggests some confusion about the impetus for new ways of moving. It may be that the term 'ballet' was being used in the way that 'dance' would be today and that the notion of new forms evolving from the one already funded was a bureaucratic imperative. The enquiry also resulted in funds being made available for commissions and bursaries, and it made recommendations about conditions of employment for dancers. The range of dance grants diversified to include education, amateur ballet clubs, notation and an increasing number of small groups. Organisations such as Balletmakers and the Association of Dance and Mime Artists were also given small grants, as were festivals.

British society also became increasingly diverse during this period. The starting point of modern immigration is generally given as the arrival of the ship, the Empire Windrush, from the West Indies in 1948. At the time there was large-scale emigration from Britain and the resultant labour shortage encouraged the Government to recruit labour from the Commonwealth. The black population of Britain doubled between 1931 and 1951, and was followed by a dramatic rise before the Commonwealth Immigration Act introduced restrictions and quotas in 1962. The incoming populations brought their own dances and their own understandings of dance. As in other areas of life, discrimination and lack of understanding created barriers for black dancers. African, Caribbean and Indian dance forms were generally regarded as exotic and were hampered by limited performance opportunities, weak marketing and lack of training provision. By the 1980s the black population was four per cent of the total British population, and the Arts Council adopted positive action strategies, including a target of spending four per cent of its grant on the arts of ethnic minorities. The Black Dance Development Trust was founded to provide information, advocacy and training, and this model was subsequently adopted by South Asian Dancers who set up their own organisation. As second and third generation Black Britons evolved different interpretations of traditional forms, however, it became increasingly difficult for umbrella organisations to encompass diverse aspirations.

Liberated notions about who could dance were central to the philosophies of New Dance and promoted by the education work of the London Contemporary Dance Theatre, which was founded on the American campus residency model. The motivation ranged between missionary zeal and the economic imperative to 'get bums on seats'. As a result more people were dancing, more vocational training courses were founded and increasing numbers of dancers emerged into a limited marketplace. In the 1970s the Manpower Services Commission (MSC) Job Creation Scheme probably did more to encourage the nationwide spread of dance than the arts funding system. For example, Ludus Dance Company received over £26 000 from MSC compared to a little over £3000 from the Arts Council and North West Arts in its first 19 months of existence. Several other regional and dance in education companies were formed in a similar way.

From 1976 another kind of dance provision emerged. It involved a dance practitioner living and working in a defined geographical area with a remit to develop dance in that area. Usually funded through a mixture of arts, education and leisure providers with local, regional and national remits, these individuals taught classes and workshops, established performance groups, promoted professional performances and residencies, raised funds, managed budgets, and provided information, advice, marketing and even catering. A few had a base with a dance studio; most were peripatetic and took dance into schools and other less likely settings, such as shopping centres, day centres and prisons. The term 'animateur' was coined to indicate a distinctive profession. As might be expected of an activity that was based on geographically isolated individuals responding to local circumstances and situations, the differences were many. There were shared high-level philosophies and objectives based on the belief that everyone can dance, that dance experience is the entitlement of everyone, and that the role of the animateur was to empower others. This had more in common with the philosophies that underpinned community arts practice than the established conventions of dance teaching. Yet, community dance was different from community arts in its ambitions for the expansion and development of the art form. Dance animateurs were concerned with promoting professional dance and with encouraging individuals to seek a professional career in dance. In the main, contemporary dance was the focus of activity. The model was successful, in part because it built on the unique strengths of dance, such as its popularity as a participatory activity and its emphasis on creating and building links between artists and communities. It laid the foundations for local and regional dance organisations, such as Regional Dance Councils, and eventually for National Dance Agencies. The 'animateur' model was subsequently adopted and promoted by other art forms, notably music and literature.

Coming of age?

By the 1970s and 1980s dance management had become vitally concerned with funding issues. The policies of the Arts Council and the Regional Arts Associations became increasingly important as a growing number and wider range of dancers sought support. A high proportion of dance activity was experimental and contemporary, and in common with all contemporary arts had limited commercial attraction. Dance was, and remains, very dependent on the arts funding system.

Necessarily, there is a relationship between the Arts Council and current government concerns. The 1980s saw a change in the way the case for the arts, specifically the case for public funding of the arts, was expressed. The Arts Council published a glossy booklet entitled *A Great British Success Story* in 1986. It made the economic case for public arts funding, talking about investment, product, achievements and national pride. Viewed from the more cynical, post-Thatcherite 1990s, some of the arguments are endearingly simple, particularly in the area of employment.

> The arts can create new jobs cheaply and, notably, create them among young people in inner city areas. As well as improving the social fabric this can bring big savings in welfare payments.
>
> Arts Council (1986)

The economic argument was based on the relationship between cost (i.e. the government grant to the arts), and income, through taxes from VAT on theatre tickets, income tax and national insurance paid by those employed in the arts (estimated at some £75 million at a time when the government grant was £106 million), and through savings on welfare benefits. Such arguments were evidently persuasive, and the following year saw an increase in the government grant to over £135 million. The eighth report of the House of Commons' Education, Science and Arts Committee on Public and Private Funding of the Arts, published in October 1982, had, to an extent, invited the argument:

> Whilst the Committee believe the funding of the arts needs no justification beyond itself we are of the opinion that the considerable economic importance of the arts is not generally appreciated by local and national government. At the simplest level, the arts represent productive employment. Whilst no firm evidence has been received by the Committee regarding the number employed in the arts, any estimate should include not only professional performers and creative artists, administrators of one kind or another and support staffs in galleries, museums, theatres, cinemas and concert halls, but also aspects of the publishing industry, broadcasting employees and workers in the film and recording industry. Thus the arts are a major industry in their own right. We estimate that the arts directly employ not less that 200,000 people, and that the turnover of the arts industry in 1981/82 approached £900,000 million.
>
> House of Commons (1982)

Thus the 'arts industry' came into being. The rationale remains pertinent. It was echoed in the National Heritage Committee's report on the funding of the Performing and Visual Arts in 1996, and is a central plank in the current Labour government's interest in the 'cultural industries'. In claiming a seat at the table of industry, the arts had to adopt a new agenda that justified funding in measurable, numerical terms. Plans, targets, performance indicators, funding agreements, formal systems of appraisal and accountability entered the funding vocabulary and became increasingly significant factors. Challenge was introduced by the Arts Council and the newly established Association for Business Sponsorship of the Arts. In 1984, the Arts Council published *The Glory of the Garden*, claiming it to be the 'first thorough and fundamental review' in the 40 years of the organisation's existence. The review aimed to be strategic, exploring the balance of funding among regions and among art forms, giving emphasis to partnerships with local authorities and the business sector and proposing a development plan. This plan was based on the expectation of growth, and it identified and costed priorities for additional funding. Dance was one such area. It was identified as underfunded, and attention was drawn to low salaries and the shortage of time and resources for new work. The main thrust of the proposals was to strengthen national touring and regionally based companies.

The company is the main structure for creating and disseminating dance as a live performing art. The relationship between companies and the environment in which they operate is crucial to their effectiveness. In the 1980s dance was rather like a railway with no stations. Companies were touring without timetables, and without 'stations' where they could refuel and where people could find out when the next train was due, where it was going and how to get on board. By the end of the 1980s, the need for a more developed dance infrastructure was clear and articulated by Graham Devlin in his report *Stepping Forward* (1989). This took a holistic view of dance, in terms of form, scale and the processes of participation, training, production and promotion. Possibly the most visible outcome of this report was the emergence of the network of National Dance Agencies which, together with a growing range of local and regional dance agencies, were to begin to provide the stations for the dance railway. Other key developments included the recognition that touring on the middle-scale was far more demanding and needed better resourcing in terms of administration and marketing; the establishment of a scheme to increase management support for emerging dance companies; and the realisation that spreading resources too thinly only served to spread the misery further.

It could be argued that the rebellion against ballet in the 1960s marked the beginning of the coming of age for dance, in that it demonstrated that dancers felt sufficiently strong to attempt to establish their own structures and ways of working. The next 20 years saw a combination of experiments with different mechanisms. Some were borrowed from established art forms: regional dance companies and dance in education companies, for example, mirrored developments in drama. Others developed from the particular qualities of dance in its contemporary forms: for instance, animateurs exploited the accessibility of participation and creation. The establishment, in the 1990s, of National Dance Agencies aimed to marry the lessons of both in recognising the local and global nature of dance, the need for stability and flexibility, and for practical support, visibility and advocacy that celebrates dance in all its diversity.

If coming of age can be marked by the confidence to rebel, then maturity is signalled by a growing awareness of the common good and a willingness to take responsibility for the community at large and the environment in which it exists. Signs of this can be found in the work of organisations such as the Foundation for Community Dance, Dance UK and the National Dance Agencies; in the crossover between dance forms and with other arts; in the collaboration of promoters to establish networks of performance opportunities; in the coming together of dance companies to push for a 'national dance house'; in the recent interest in mentoring; and in the enduring influence of the writings of Peter Brinson.[1]

A sense of direction?

This may seem a long way from the contemporary concerns of the dance manager. Understanding how we got here does not necessarily help determine where we are going. Yet the job of the dance manager has been shaped by a particular history and is determined by the prevailing climate. Understanding this may at least help to maintain the sanity of the individual manager who is faced with a complex array of quasi-commercial tasks in the relatively chaotic, creative atmosphere that prevails in many dance organisations. The range of organisations contains its own array of paradoxes. The largest may be hierarchical in structure and bureaucratic in operation, the smallest may be dominated by the personality of the artistic leader. The apparently conflicting demands of accountability and creativity have to be reconciled in the person of the dance manager.

While the future may not be predictable, it is certain to bring further change. To an extent, the business of dance is ahead of the business of business. The uncertainties that are rocking the large industrial and commercial institutions have never been certainties for dance, where jobs have always been precarious and career paths fragmented. The concern with adopting the language and practices of business that flowed from the policies of the 1980s brought benefits, not the least in professionalising the role of the dance manager. The disadvantage was that it also brought distraction and loss of confidence. It may be that another phase is dawning. Writers such as Charles Handy and Will Hutton are arguing for a more holistic view of economics that takes account of the personal and social costs and encourages a 'good' society. Hutton (1995) argues for a 'moral economy'; Handy sees opportunity in the end of employment as it has been understood throughout the century:

> Britain will never be 'Great' again, in the sense that she could be a world power or an economic force again, but she could find a new cause and forge a new existence as, for instance, the 'Athens of Europe', meaning the old Athens of learning, culture and the arts. Her great comparative advantage is her language. Everyone, every-where, wants to learn it. Her universities, theatres, designers, artists, architects, film and TV makers, writers and literati, musicians and dancers are world-class. Sadly, she is more likely to be known as a

museum than a cultural centre, but the opportunity is there to . . .lift her people, to give her a sense of new direction.

Handy (1994, p.266)

It is, perhaps, another sign of change that it is economists who are beginning to assert values and qualities beyond sheer numbers, and the popularity of their books suggests they are finding resonance with the experiences and concerns of many.

Dance as a contemporary art form will always be dependent on a mixed economy. The dance audience is buying experience rather than something tangible. Frequently, that experience is challenging rather than comforting. These qualities may find resonance with the next phase, but it is unlikely to be sufficient to remove dance from the need for some form of funding.

The story of dance in twentieth-century Britain is one of establishing structures and organisations. Without these it is unlikely that there would be the diversity of forms, styles and approaches that are available today. Because of these developments the job of the dance manager is more formalised, but still requires entrepreneurial flair. A larger number of companies has brought a higher profile to the art form, but has increased competition for funds and bookings among companies. The manager of the independent dance artist or company needs to be skilled in finance, marketing, audience development, booking tours, and contracts, and to understand a wide range of legal and fiscal procedures. Above all, however, dance is a people industry. The dance manager needs to be committed to the artist and their vision, adept at dealing with people and their egos, to build permanent and temporary teams, and to communicate with a wide range of people in a variety of situations. The people, products and peculiarities of dance distinguish it from other management contexts, and provide both the greatest frustration and the greatest reward for dance managers.

End notes

1. Peter Brinson described himself as a dance politician and was influential in articulating the concerns common to all dancers, thereby pulling together a disparate profession, and in winning respectability and a place for dance in the context of the wider educational, social and political agendas. He died in 1995.

References

Arnold-Baker, C. (1983), *Practical Law for Administrators*, London: John Offord.
Arts Council of Great Britain (1986) *A Great British Success Story*, London: Arts

Council.

Baldry, H. (1981) *The Case for the Arts*, London: Secker & Warburg.

Coton, A. V. (1975) *Writings on Dance 1938–68*, London: Dance Books.

Devlin, G. (1989) *Stepping Forward*, London: The Arts Council of Great Britain.

DiMaggio, P. (1991) 'Cultural Entrepreneurship in Nineteenth-Century Boston: the Creation of an Organisational Base for High Culture in America', in Mukerji C. & Schudson, M., *Rethinking Popular Culture: Contemporary Perspectives in Cultural Studies*, California: University of California Press. See also *Media, Culture and Society* (1982), London: Sage.

Galbraith, J.K. (1987), in Trevor May, *An Economic and Social History of Britain 1760–1970*, London: Longman.

Grigorovich, S.L. (1953) *The Diaghilev Ballet 1909–1929*, London: Constable.

Handy, C. (1994) *The Empty Raincoat*, London: Arrow Books.

Haskell, A. (1944) *The National Ballet: a History and a Manifesto*, London: Adam & Charles Black.

House of Commons (1982) *Eighth Report of the House of Commons' Education, Science and Arts Committee on Public and Private Funding of the Arts*.

Hutton, W. (1995) *The State We're In*, London: Jonathon Cape.

Jenkins, H. (1979) *The Culture Gap: an Experiment of the Government and the Arts 1974–1976*, London: Marion Boyars.

Mackrell, J. (1992) *Out of Line: the Story of British New Dance*, London: Dance Books.

May, T. (1987) *An Economic and Social History of Britain 1790–1970*, London: Longman.

Pick, J. (1983) T*he West End: Mismanagement and Snobbery*, London: John Afford.

White, E. (1975) *The Arts Council of Great Britain*, London: Davis Poynter.

White, J. (ed) (1985) *Twentieth-Century Dance in Britain*, London: Dance Books.

MANAGING DANCE ARTISTS

Introduction

Linda Jasper

Dance is a people business, dependent on a unique blend of individuals with different skills and perspectives. Relationships between artists and managers are notoriously complex. Julia Carruthers opens Chapter 3 by quoting a significant relationship for dance, that between Nijinsky and Diaghilev, which eventually failed. How can the seemingly incompatible functions of the artist creating works to satisfy his or her own needs and the manager operating in an open market place be reconciled? Most artists, whatever the size of their companies or the genre of dance in which they work, realise that they need assistance to manage their work, as Kari O'Nions's research proves (Chapter 2). Both O'Nions and Carruthers make it clear that the relationship between manager and artist is of utmost importance.

In addition to sustaining an empathetic and good relationship with the artist, the manager is also engaged in other challenges. Managing change generated from external forces, such as funding bodies and venues, and the unpredictable nature of the artistic process itself, create significant pressure for administrators. In the fluctuating and competitive arts world both artists and managers agree that, in order for dance to survive, 'hard' skills are needed, particularly in the areas of fund-raising and marketing. Carruthers explains that dedication to the artists' creative practice sustains managers who work in this taxing and under-resourced industry. The individuals identified primarily as creative are artists, but it quickly becomes apparent that a broader understanding of creativity is needed to encompass the dance manager. Managers such as Carruthers, and the artists interviewed in O'Nions's chapter, are searching for a wider support base, whether through mentoring from peers, advice from other administrators, or backing from members of the artistic team and the board. Clearly there is a need for managers to retain their own identity when taking on the role of managing creative artists, and it is vital that their needs are met through interesting work and career progression.

The scale of operation and nature of the product also has an effect on how the artistic process is managed. O'Nions suggests that the size of the company produces different management styles. Carruthers, reporting on the management of a medium-scale, cutting edge contemporary dance company, illustrates the fluid way of working between artistic director and manager, which O'Nions describes as typical at this scale.

Selling British contemporary dance to venues in other European countries is sometimes easier than it is in the United Kingdom. Carruthers has built profitable relationships with a range of promoters on the continent. Guy Cools, the dance programmer at the Vooruit Arts Centre in Gent, Belgium, is one such contact. He discusses a model of working that demands a high level of understanding of the needs of the artist, and he describes his role as an interpreter of this to the wider world. Speaking directly to artists, as a promoter, he emphasises the need of the artist to have access to adequate time and space for the extended creative process. He suggests that artists must be in control of how their work is managed, produced and presented: this, he argues, is a fundamental part of the creative process. He sees his role as helping artists to translate their needs in a political and economic context. There is, however, a danger that the translation process may distort the aims of the artistic product, therefore Cools insists that artists have a responsibility to understand and take charge of this process.

O'Nions argues that management models cannot be transferred from one situation to another, as each artist requires a different way of working, but principles can. These should be based on an empathetic professional working relationship where artists and managers share a core purpose and vision for the work and, ideally, should acknowledge the creative role that managers play in realising the artistic ambitions of the artists for whom they work.

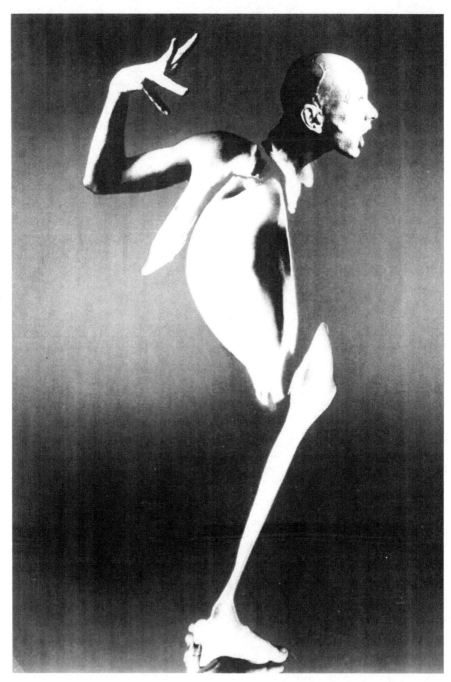

Photo: Gary Clark/Matthew Hawker
Wayne MacGregor, Random Dance Company

2

How Choreographers Want to be Managed

Kari O'Nions

I think it's about respecting individual artist's choices, more than trying to institutionalise an idea.

Thus spoke Random Dance Company's artistic director, Wayne McGregor,[1] discussing approaches to managing choreographers during a recent interview. His are wise and pertinent words. McGregor was just one of seven choreographers who contributed to the research undertaken for this chapter. The focus of this work is an examination, based on extensive interview material, into how choreographers want to be managed. The research revealed both incredible congruency and disparity of opinion among the choreographers to the various questions posed during research interviews. The need, to use McGregor's own words, for 'respecting individual artist's choices' and carefully taking on board individual's needs and contexts, as well as avoiding 'blanket approaches' to managing choreographers, became crystal clear.

In the management of choreographers, it is crucial that ideas are not 'institutionalised', particularly in the current climate of 'discontinuous' change. As we approach the new millennium, the context in which choreographers are managing and being managed is increasingly complex and altering rapidly: for example, with the recent advent of lottery funding, numerous funding body and client reviews, and the pressure to take a more business-like approach to the arts. It is a time when there is often little time. Consequently, there is a temptation to re-adopt familiar 'tried and tested' methods that may no longer be appropriate in a new, ever-changing context. The successful development of dance management practice, and its integration with more 'formal' business management procedures, has the potential to fail or succeed, depending partly on the quantity and quality of consideration given to the real needs of the choreographer. These actual, stated needs are therefore the focus of this chapter.

In exploring the choreographers' perspective here, it is readily acknowledged that this focus is but one side of the coin, or rather of a multi-faceted diamond. There are, of course, other perspectives: those of managers, consultants, funders and the paying public, to name a few, some of which are impressively explored in other chapters of this book. Dance management, however, must first and foremost, as McGregor says, be about 'respecting individual artist's choices', and hence the choreographer's opinion is taken as the starting point for exploration.

Research methodology

The research itself explores a number of key issues and questions in relation to the concept of 'dance management': the appropriateness of the term 'manager'; the skills and qualities valued in a dance manager; the choreographer's ideal or dream situation; the notion of 'control' and where it lies; the choreographer/manager relationship; and the potential realisation of a choreographer's artistic vision.

These are some of the issues raised during extensive interviews with seven contemporary British choreographers: Wayne McGregor of Random Dance Company; David Bintley[2] of Birmingham Royal Ballet; George Dzikunu[3] of Adzido Pan African Dance Ensemble; Rosemary Butcher;[4] Paula Hampson[6] of Paula Hampson Dance Company; Shobana Jeyasingh[6] of Shobana Jeyasingh Dance Company; and Mark Murphy[7] of V-Tol Dance Company. This sample was chosen to provide a range of British choreographers at various stages of their career, working at varying company scales and across a diversity of dance styles. All of the choreographers interviewed are publicly funded, although some also work in the commercial sector.

Interviews contributing to this research were conducted either face-to-face or via telephone during 1997 and early 1998, and ranged from 20 minutes to over an hour in length. Pertinent issues and questions were identified before the interviews commenced, but interviews were then loosely structured to avoid, as far as possible, any line of questioning that would predetermine or direct the interviewees' responses, and to encourage the choreographers to speak in their own words.

The following key questions were asked:

- How do choreographers feel about themselves and their companies being managed?
- What are the skills and qualities required of a good manager?
- Is the role of dance manager an unrewarding one?
- What would be your 'dream management' scenario?
- How is the artistic/management relationship controlled?
- What are the obstacles to achieving artistic vision?

THE RESEARCH FINDINGS

Being managed

How do choreographers feel about themselves and their companies being managed? 'Yes. I definitely need to be managed', said Mark Murphy clearly, 'I know that I can't do it all on my own.' Likewise George Dzikunu acknowledged a definite need for management: 'I think you need a manager to manage every artist – otherwise things get out of control.' Murphy and Dzikunu echoed the general consensus of those interviewed that some kind of management was necessary and useful for a choreographer.

Yet what was meant by 'some kind of management'? No one single definition of management was suggested to the interviewees, but the term was left open to interpretation. As expected, the choreographers, partially due to their differing contexts and company scales, interpreted the term 'management' differently. Under the rubric of 'manager', the interviewees included: administrators, company managers, administrative directors, agents, mentors, the company's executive committee, the board, and the Arts Council of England. The focus of most discussion, however, was upon the role of administrators, general managers and administrative directors.

Only one choreographer interviewed doubted whether she required any form of management: 'I wouldn't want to be under continual management because I think that, unless the person absolutely relates to who you are and what you are, you can be pushed in different directions . . . It's very much about people coming in and thinking they are in control. I refuse to be controlled.'

This choreographer was more convinced (although still not wholly) of the usefulness of a personal assistant, rather than a manager or administrator. Occasionally, then, the terms 'management' and 'manager' may, for some choreographers, confer too much ownership of the artistic product and the administrative function upon that manager. This is more likely to happen with choreographers working at small- and middle-scale, rather than in large-scale companies.

Managers' skills and qualities

What are the skills and qualities required of a good manager? Here the choreographers were significantly more concerned with the manager's personal qualities and personality than with his or her actual administrative skills. The administrative skills required are clearly dependent upon company scale: they might range from reception duties, travel, accommodation and tour booking to financial management and co-ordinating education work; or from marketing, fund-raising and sponsorship to strategy-making and advocacy. Requirements in terms of administrative skills were, as would be expected, extremely variable.

Paula Hampson, a choreographer in the early stages of her career (who at the time of being interviewed was about to commence working, for the first time, with an administrator one day a week) was concerned with getting 'help with making applications and getting them in on time' and with 'organising teaching schedules and programmes of work'. In contrast, according to David Bintley, the administrative director for Birmingham Royal Ballet is responsible for 'the whole of the administration, and the orchestra and physiotherapy department, and contracts with dancers, to name a few'.

In describing the qualities of a manager, there was a surprising congruency of opinion from choreographers across company scale. Words such as 'empathy', 'sympathy', 'understanding', 'appreciation' and 'trust' recurred frequently in interviews. For Shobana Jeyasingh, 'the most important thing is to get someone who is in sympathy with whatever you want to do. The commitment to the work is the most important', she said, 'because you can learn to be a first-class administrator, if you have the right motivation, but you cannot learn to be committed'.

The choreographers also overwhelmingly emphasised the need for a good interpersonal relationship with their manager. Hampson, for example, suggested that there would need to be 'some kind of wavelength, some kind of meeting point'. Rosemary Butcher discussed the need for 'someone who likes me and doesn't undermine me', since 'if you have a relationship day in day out over your work which is not a positive one, it really, really undermines you'. She also requested 'someone who is really able to work with me and my particular life and understanding, strong but not over dominant. I suppose in a way I want someone where there isn't any ego'.

Another crucial factor was good communication skills. Wayne McGregor mentioned the need for someone 'who really listens', adding: 'it's vital for me to have a dialogue, and a dialogue of a level which can be challenged'. A need for the manager to have a clear understanding of the choreographer's thinking and intellectual direction is evidently important. At all scales, a lack of clear communication was cited as a key factor in the failure of the choreographer/manager relationship. It is perhaps when the negotiation and discussion is replaced by non-communication that failure is imminent. As Dzikunu said: 'If there is frequent communication between the artistic person and the manager, I don't think much should go wrong'.

Equally important for the choreographers was being managed by someone who understood, or even had a personal experience of, dance. Bintley repeatedly acknowledged the benefits to be gained from the fact that

Birmingham Royal Ballet's administrative director was once a dancer: 'It gives him an added insight which is vitally important. He's not just a banker or somebody holding the purse strings, so he really appreciates what we are trying to do, and necessity of finding the money from somewhere.'

If a potential manager does not have this personal dance experience, Dzikunu suggested that he or she should have some form of induction to aid understanding: 'When you are dealing with artists, you have really got to understand their ups and downs. I think the main thing I would like a manager to have is an experience of being an artist . . . to have a little bit of training or an induction, a way to be able to understand. If you just bring in a manager from the commercial sector, the understanding of being an artist is always a difficulty.'

To summarise from the interviewees' various requirements of the ideal manager listed thus far, the composite specification of a good manager might read as follows:

- non-egotistical
- sympathetic and empathic
- good interpersonal and communication skills
- a clear understanding, if not personal experience of, dance and the choreographers' direction
- trustworthy
- committed
- non-undermining.

Among the other requests or requirements for our ideal manager were 'loyalty', 'decision making abilities', 'dedication', 'trust' and, to top it all, 'a thick skin'.

Dance manager: an unrewarding role?

Interestingly, several choreographers expressed voluntary concern over the managerial role, admitting it was no easy task. Murphy, for example, suggested that it was 'the most thankless job, and also the hardest, in that there isn't a lot of pay off; [the manager is] left sorting out problems that are a pain in the neck'.

The choreographers also emphasised and empathised with the lack of career development for the manager. Jeyasingh and Dzikunu both discussed the problem of managers leaving the company after a couple of years. For Dzikunu: 'We advertise, they start work, it takes time to make the person feel what you are doing, and by the time that has happened, the person is moving on again.' According to Jeyasingh, 'people reach a particular level and actually they can't learn any more, and there's nowhere for them to go, so they go to work for a venue, a public institution or become freelance consultants'.

'There's a real dearth of jobs at the top end of the management spectrum', Jeyasingh continued:

> You can be director of Dance Umbrella, but there aren't that many Dance Umbrellas! The dance community is a very small one and therefore it's difficult for people to keep on learning. Also, it's such hard work, people just get burnt out. I myself can't see what you do after six years or so... Once you run a middle-scale, choreographer-led company, or a choreographer's company, the choreographer personally might be continually learning new things, but for the administrator, it's probably a kind of repeat.

According to choreographers then, there is scope for improving the career progression of their managers. There may be hope for our 'ideal composite manager' yet.

The dream management scenario

Hitherto discussed has been the ideal manager, but if, in an ideal world, a choreographer could have anything at all in terms of management – a dream management situation – what would it be?

Some choreographers, like Murphy, were more immediately concerned with improving the company's financial situation and material resources. 'A dream situation would be to have more management staff in the company like the current staff', he said, 'and, without being greedy, to be in a much more comfortable situation financially. I'll take care of the artistic side as long as somebody else, or a group of people, take care of that.' Other interviewees were more interested in gaining support in artistic and choreographic development. Hampson discussed the benefits of an artistic mentor who would be 'someone who knew your work and your history so well, that you could bounce ideas off, someone guiding you.. someone to get feedback from...add another voice'.

McGregor, who had already engineered mentoring opportunities with British choreographers such as Richard Alston and Shobana Jeyasingh, was very clear on the benefits of this way of working:

> It's really vital. It's a real tragedy that we don't have more of it in this country. It really disappoints me that you have senior artists...who never get the chance to dialogue with younger choreographers...that

dialogue is an absolutely vital one that can push your thinking through the roof.

'I'd like to see something like a choreographic centre (where money is really taken totally out of the equation deliberately which is obviously very difficult)', continued McGregor, 'where everybody very openly and in an honest way responds to each other as choreographers. I would love, although I'd find it difficult as well, to hear truthfully what people think about my work and really push that dialogue. We should also be sharing resources and models of practice much more.'

Likewise, Bintley recognised the need for more artistic guidance in his younger self: 'I probably wouldn't have liked it much at the time, but it would have been good for me and it would have saved me some blushes...things that I really should have been warned against!' Because of this, at Birmingham Royal Ballet, Bintley has instigated a choreographic scheme that he personally mentors, where young dancers in the company work together to create ballets, choreographing in small groups, for performance.

For Dzikunu, research and development requires communication with choreographers in Africa, and therefore being able to fund travel is vital:

> In terms of having other people to help with artistic thinking, there haven't always been a lot of people around here that have the same situation, so it has been difficult. I bounce ideas when I travel to Africa, to meet other choreographers, I get my strength when I travel there. But even if I wasn't able to travel more, I would love to be able bring people over here to give seminars to share ideas with others.

The emphasis in the choreographers' responses to imagining a dream management situation is focused notably upon support in creating the artistic product, through mentoring and dialogue with other choreographers, as well as on increased management or administrative support.

Artistic and management control and the artistic/management relationship

The issues of control, and maximising the choreographer's potential for realising the artistic vision, were ones which also concerned many choreographers. '[The company's vision] is definitely my vision, and I feel very much ownership of that vision', said McGregor, for whom a manager was someone who buys into the company's artistic vision: 'Someone who wants to realise that vision...who wants to share it, and push it further.' Jeyasingh echoed McGregor's opinions: 'It's all to do with artistic policy and vision, rather than necessarily always doing what is the most expedient.' Dzikunu agreed: 'In terms of control, the full control should lie with the artistic person, because it is an artistic company.'

There was a general consensus that the choreographer should have artistic control, but what about the control of the administrative or management function? While some choreographers felt that the control they desired over the company's administrative resources was fluid and flexible depending on the context, others were very clear of their need for ultimate management control. Notably, some choreographers performed certain activities which are more commonly associated with the manager's role, themselves: fund-raising and liaising with funders; tour, travel and accommodation booking; or finding performance spaces.

If a manager is over-dominant, according to Butcher, then the choreographer's position is weakened: 'I don't mind people saying "you should try this or that", but the reversal of that is when you are put in the very weak situation of not being able to fulfil your legacy and that is vicious.' When asked whether an administrator or manager would have any control over her work at all, Butcher replied, 'absolutely not'. For Murphy, artistic director of a middle-scale company, the degree of choreographer's control is a variable: 'It changes. It's much more about the relationship; you are sometimes contained, and sometimes not contained.' McGregor explained that he is 'very creative about administration...I don't see it as solely the managers' responsibility...I've always found it useful to go to funding meetings and meetings with sponsors.'

This fluid interrelationship between the artist and the management within a company seemed most apparent at middle-scale. Just as choreographers had input into administrative decision making, in some cases the management had involvement in the artistic decision-making. 'I view the company as a whole and I try to instil a sense that everybody has a say in everything, so I would sometimes ask Susanne [V-Tol Dance Company's General Manager], or other people I trust, to comment in a rehearsal', said Murphy. According to Jeyasingh, also artistic director of a middle-scale company:

> In a way, you cannot separate out the two because the person who manages your budget, in some ways, manages the artistic and the way you divide up your resources will in some ways depend on what you want to do.

With Birmingham Royal Ballet, a large-scale company, there seemed to be a clearer delineation between the artistic and administrative sides of the company, with an artistic director as well as an administrative director. When asked whether the administrative director ever supported the artistic director in artistic decision-making, Bintley explained: 'Whilst the administrative director shares the artistic vision, and will defend it on all grounds, not only financially, in terms of artistic decision-making, as he rightly says, that is not really his position. He can only say what he likes and dislikes.'

As already mentioned, Birmingham Royal Ballet's administrative director has, according to Bintley, wide-ranging responsibilities. While Bintley, like McGregor, is involved in fundraising, he adds: 'I am really only in charge of the dancers and the ballet staff... well, I say only, there are 80 of them! I would say that an organisation this size is a business. So I see the administrative director as my equal.'

Realising the artistic vision

Both implicitly and explicitly, in many choreographers' comments, there is a unanimous concern with the ultimate protection of the artistic vision. This suggests that, in addition to the aforementioned qualities, a good manager would also wholeheartedly be invested in the choreographer's vision and most gainfully employed more often in a supportive and facilitative role, and less often in a directive one. Given the choreographers' obvious concern with maximising their potential to realise their artistic vision, this begs the question of what, in the choreographers' opinion, has disallowed this previously.

Dzikunu, artistic director of a large-scale company, admitted that he has felt pressure from time to time to do what is financially expedient rather than what is in line with his artistic policy:

> I think there has been pressure on me sometimes; it comes once in a while and then goes again. I bring in different freelance directors; they might come with different ideas for making the whole thing commercial, or going to the West End, and there you are obviously going to lose certain things, your artistic qualities. The research of doing traditional African dance has been the main thing for the company, and I wouldn't want to water that down for the sake of moving to the West End.

Bintley also admitted to challenges: 'We have to make huge efforts on every piece that we do now to try and get some kind of private sponsorship. We have to jump through hoops, write out proposals and convince bankers and business men that this is the most exciting thing they have ever seen . . . again!'

On a more positive note, according to Bintley, these obstacles to realising the artistic vision are surmountable through creative thinking:

> It's a question of balance. If you can produce some work which is going to put proverbial bums on seats, and can produce some work that is going to secure money, then you can afford to take some risks. What I am trying to do is excite people with risk. It is something that large ballet companies have shied away from for a long time, and putting new ballet on any programme became box office poison.

With staff invested in his risk-taking vision, Bintley believes that the company can afford to take risks successfully: 'It really is the case for the whole company, from the orchestra to the press office, that they are excited about doing new work. I think everybody realises with a bit more effort, that danger and risk is much more exciting than doing a better deal – which everybody has done. But to make history is exciting.'

The potential for realising the artistic vision for upcoming choreographers may be similarly hampered through lack of resources, but this time the potential absence of little or no administrative assistance whatsoever is making life very hard. 'All the applications I have done', admits Hampson, 'have been panic, mayhem, last minute, faxing things everywhere, staying up until 5 o'clock in the morning. It's not the right way to do things.'

It may be that life is slightly easier for choreographers working at middle-scale rather than small-scale, where there is little or no management support, as Hampson described, or at large-scale, where there are pressures to commercialise, as Dzikunu highlighted. Certainly, there was less concern expressed among choreographers at middle-scale, than those at small- and large-scale. As Jeyasingh, artistic director of a middle-scale company, said: 'For the artist, finally, it's a question of the area they want to work in. You may not want to be another Royal Ballet.'

CONCLUSIONS

To summarise, most choreographers deeply value some form of management but, for some choreographers, this term confers too much ownership on the artistic product. When considering the qualities and skills of an ideal manager, many choreographers emphasised the personal qualities rather than the administrative skill-base of that manager: they required an empathetic, loyal, committed individual, who has a clear understanding of dance and the artistic direction and vision of the company. The choreographers also voluntarily expressed concern over the managerial role being occasionally unrewarding and non-developmental.

As revealed by the very differing needs described by each choreographer, individual requirements must be carefully considered. These may be based upon a choreographer's particular artistic vision and direction, company scale, the current level of financial and management support, the choreographer's personal level of administrative input and knowledge, the choreographer's need or desire for public recognition or fame, and his or her personality, to name only a few.

On considering a dream management situation, there was a surprising emphasis upon the desire for support in the creation of the artistic product (rather than management/administrative support) that might be gained through mentoring, as McGregor suggested, or through seminars, as Dzikunu mentioned. Coincidentally, there was a concern among choreographers to retain artistic control and to maximise the potential for realising the artistic vision, which seemed generally less problematic at middle-scale, although further research would be required before drawing too many conclusions. The choreographers' degree and level of management control varied considerably, again partly depending upon company scale.

The route ahead?

While once more emphasising the importance of considering each choreographer's case individually, it may be helpful to draw together some initial suggestions for the development of best dance management practice, based on the findings, many of which could be implemented by choreographers and managers themselves. Given that the needs of choreographers clearly differ, the importance of choreographers themselves being totally clear on management criteria becomes paramount. It is essential that choreographers take time, and are given time, to consider and be realistic about their management requirements, and of course these requirements will change over time. If these requirements are not clear for choreographers, it may be worth companies investing in internal or external consultancies to look at the choreographers' needs: these should then be given full consideration when appointing new management staff.

In inducting new staff, adequate consideration should be given to team building, given the clear importance of the interpersonal relationship between choreographer and management staff, revealed in the interviews. Since the need for understanding of dance was mentioned by several interviewees, it may be worthwhile, as Dzikunu suggested, organising induction in practical dance understanding for staff who do not have the first-hand practical dance experience that Bintley valued so highly.

41

If, as has been seen, a high level of investment in the artistic vision is required from a manager, then it is critical that the choreographer takes time to find ways to communicate this vision effectively to management staff. Researching ways of investing all staff in that vision (as with the situation Bintley described at Birmingham Royal Ballet), through choreographers and companies sharing advice and information on ways of achieving this, may prove beneficial. It could be something as simple as valuing the management's opinions over artistic decision-making and instilling 'a sense that everybody has a say in everything', as Murphy described. Proper consideration into ways of ensuring team investment in the artistic vision may further enable the appropriate understanding and empathy in the artistic vision described by choreographers as valuable qualities in a manager.

As there is a clear concern from choreographers over the manager's job satisfaction, and coincidentally several interviewees discussed problems resulting from a high management staff turnover, it may be worthwhile for companies and choreographers to increase their consideration of how the choreographers' career development can be paralleled by their managers. Companies, choreographers, managers and funding bodies that invest more in the manager's training and career development, or indeed help managers to resource their own training, may alleviate the high staff turnover and resulting lost expertise and time spent on repeated inductions.

Finally, given the clear interest from choreographers in gaining greater artistic support, particularly through mentoring, it would be beneficial to consider further ways of developing choreographers' artistic development. Schemes are already under way, either self-resourced by choreographers, like McGregor described, or based on previous experience, like Bintley's scheme at Birmingham Royal Ballet. McGregor talked about sharing resources with younger choreographers, and this may be a useful model for future exploration. Various methods of facilitating the communication between choreographers, like McGregor's notion of a choreographic centre, might also be further considered.

The interviews have already revealed some very clear successes in dance management practice, from choreographers facilitating their own mentoring and setting up schemes for younger choreographers, to choreographers working towards investing their team in their artistic vision. Choreographers are clear on their need for management, and are generally appreciative of the experience, commitment, organisational capabilities of, and hard work undertaken by, managers, as well as the challenges they face. Choreographers are keen to find ways to facilitate their own, as well as their managers', development. It is crucial to believe in, build on, and continually disseminate the models of good practice already occurring. As Charles Handy (1995) says in *What Show Business Can Show Business*:

> Sometimes management suffers from an excess of rationality, an overdose of the familiar, an obsession with tidiness, and a belief that money will solve everything. It is well to be reminded that there are other ways of making things happen, and that a round of applause can mean much more than a cheque, and that it is possible for ordinary people to make magic if they care enough about what they are doing.

The skilled dance manager has a good deal to offer. He or she necessarily undertakes a committed, creative, supportive, facilitative, interpersonally skilled, and even selfless or invisible management style that continually maximises limited resources.

Principles of Good Dance Management

- To respect individual choreographers' differing needs
- To allow the realisation of the choreographers' artistic vision through sound artistic, as well as management, support
- To facilitate clear communication between choreographer and manager
- To take into account both the choreographers' and the managers' career development
- To learn appropriately and selectively from other management practices

---

By continuing to develop, communicate, and disseminate good practice, it may be, as Handy suggests, that dance managers can teach big business a thing or two!

Kari O'Nions sincerely thanks all the choreographers who gave up their time to be interviewed for her research.

Notes

1. Wayne McGregor is artistic director of Random Dance Company. He studied at University College Bretton Hall and New York's José Limón School before founding 'Random' in 1992. Today the company has a national and international reputation, is a resident company at The Place in London, and is a past recipient of a *Time Out* nomination. McGregor, who was the recipient of the 1998 Prix d'auteur du conseil general de Seine Saint-Denis, has choreographed for companies such as Italy's Olympic Ballet and British Ricochet Dance Company, for the English National Opera and the Scottish National Opera. Film work includes Martin Sherman's *Bent*, starring Ian McKellan and Mick Jagger.

2. David Bintley became director of Birmingham Royal Ballet in 1995, succeeding Peter Wright, and has since created *Carmina Burana, The Nutcracker Sweetie, Far From the Madding Crowd* and *Edward II* for the company. His career began with Sadler's Wells Royal Ballet in 1976, and in 1978 he created *The Outsider*, his first professional work for the company. In 1983 he was appointed Company Choreographer at Sadler's Wells Royal Ballet, and in 1986 transferred to The Royal Ballet where he was Resident Choreographer until 1993. Bintley's ballets are in the repertoire of companies in America, Canada, Germany and South Africa.

3. George Dzikunu is artistic director of Adzido Pan African Dance Ensemble. Born in Ghana, and coming from a family of master drummers of the Anlo tribe in the Volta region, dancing and drumming formed an intrinsic part of his life from an early age. In Ghana, Dzikunu worked with prominent groups such as the African Theatre Troupe and the Ghana National Dance Ensemble; and formed the Sankofa Dance Company, which toured to Great Britain where Dzikunu subsequently decided to settle. He founded Adzido Pan African Dance Ensemble in 1984 initially to train people in the skills of African dance and drumming. The opportunity arose for George to direct *In the Village of Africa* and this commission enabled the formation of Adzido 12 in 1987. Revenue funding in 1990 enables the growth and development of the large-scale company, Adzido Pan African Dance Ensemble, which has now grown into the largest African dance company in Europe.

4. Rosemary Butcher is artistic director of Rosemary Butcher Dance Company. She trained at Dartington College of Arts in 1965, before visiting the US in 1969 and 1970–72 to broaden her training and study with Judson Dance Theater. Returning to Britain, she made her first choreography in 1974, called *Uneven Time*, and formed her own company the following year. The company made its first appearance at the Serpentine Gallery in 1976, and gradually built a firm audience following over the years. One of Butcher's best known works is *Touch the Earth* (1987), based on a book of photographs and writings of the same name, which was performed at the Queen Elizabeth Hall, and also televised by the BBC. Teaching and lecturing has always been an important adjunct to Butcher's choreographic work, and she has lectured during her career at Dunfermline College, Dartington College, and more recently at the University of

Surrey and the Laban Centre for Movement and Dance.

5. Paula Hampson is an independent dance performer, teacher and choreographer, based in the North West of England. As a performer she has worked with companies and artists such as the Gregory Nash Group, Maclennan Dance & Company, Julyen Hamilton and Small Bones Dance Company. As well as teaching throughout the UK in further education colleges, schools, arts centres, and dance organisations, she is becoming an increasingly well-established choreographer whose work has received support from North-West Arts Board, Arts Council of England, Suffolk Dance and The Princess Trust, to name a few.

6. Shobana Jeyasingh (artistic director and choreographer) has directed the Shobana Jeyasingh Dance Company since 1988. During the past ten years she and her company have been awarded three Digital Dance Awards and the prestigious Prudential Award for the Arts. Jeyasingh's work for the theatre includes *Cyrano* at the Royal National Theatre and her television work includes *Duet With Automobiles* for BBC2, which was shortlisted for the IMZ Dance Screen Award. The company is also the subject of a BBC2 documentary *In Between*, screened in 1997. In 1996 *Palimpsest* was awarded the Time Out dance award for best choreography. In 1995 Shobana Jeyasingh was awarded an MBE, an Honorary Doctorate from de Montfort University and an Honorary Masters Degree from the University of Surrey.

7. Mark Murphy is artistic director of V-Tol Dance Company which he formed in 1991. Graduating from the Laban Centre in 1989, the following year Murphy won a London Dance & Performance Award. His first work for V-Tol was *Crash and Burn* for the company's debut at The Place Theatre. The winner of a British New Choreography Award (1994) and a Wingate Scholarship, Murphy has also created dance films for V-Tol, as well as creating work for other companies such as National Youth Dance Company and Edinburgh's Dance Productions. He has worked as movement director for Northern Stage Company and Caryl Churchill's play *Blue Heart*.

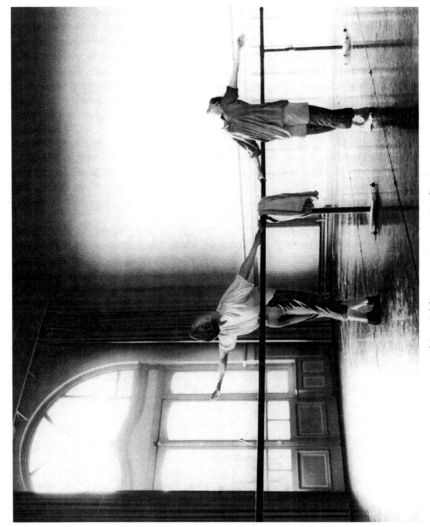

Joachim Schlömen at Dance Studio 1.

3

Managing Artists

Julia Carruthers

Sergei Diaghilev was a shrewd, sophisticated, intelligent man; in comparison Nijinsky was a simple youth...Both had motives for using one another, and in the end both felt betrayed and exploited.

MacMillan in Nijinsky (1991)

Steinhoff: The artists need a kind of partner; they don't need a slave. They always want a slave...They want to have somebody who is solving their problems, helping them in being successful, who they can treat like they want. The main piece of advice I can give to people coming into my profession is to fight against this tendency of your artistic partner to make you a slave – in his own interest!

Forsythe: We've been a team. We have a great understanding and patience with each other...and that's the secret. I couldn't do this job without him. He protects us.

William Forsythe (Artistic Director) and Herr Dr Martin Steinhoff (General Director) of Frankfurt Ballet (1997)

Choreographers and dancers cannot and do not work alone. Poets and painters toiling away in solitary confinement can be disorganised, but creating and performing in dance is about collaboration. Planning, scheduling, being on time and communicating with others are all essential to the process of making and presenting dance. Without management and subtle administration paying attention to the details, for dance, it is impossible to get the show on, to tour, find an audience and to sustain a livelihood. The partnership between creative artist and supportive, tactical administrator is vital.

Pioneers in a demoralising landscape

Too often dance seems to wallow in the low status of the art form and poor self-esteem. There have been few, if any, household names; press and

47

television coverage is scarce and those involved in dance regularly bewail the lack of 'motor-mouthed' champions for the art form. If you work as a dance manager hardly anybody has heard of the artists you have temporarily committed your life to. Salaries are rare and pay is low, especially compared to remuneration for similar work in the commercial sector. The subsidised arts lack the glamour and importance which is an accepted part of film or television. This backdrop can be demoralising, even if it leaves you feeling that you have pioneering integrity.

Dance management can be a lonely business, particularly for administrators working for smaller companies. They often work alone in an office space miles away from where the company are rehearsing and seldom see the artistic director and dancers; meetings are snatched in tea shops or on the edge of the studio at the end of the performing company's working day, when artists are sweaty and tired. It is generally the manager who is least acknowledged and applauded, and who hovers selflessly as the tired and anxious looking figure. The fact that managers are responsible for finding the money to realise projects and being the brainchild behind big developments goes unremarked. Managers are not toiling long hours for themselves or for their own glory, nor do they see themselves as charismatic showstoppers. In many cases (for example in the choreographer-led companies) without the artistic director making the work, the company would not exist, but the manager is replaceable; his or her job can be advertised and somebody else found. Yet, nonetheless, managers are cornered into feeling indispensable. How could they ever leave the job when the whole operation is so reliant on them and their specialist knowledge and contacts, painstakingly built up over many years?

Distinguishing features of the dance manager

Anyone conducting market research on dance managers in England would instantly observe that there is a sex bias in favour of women: a 'monstrous regiment'. Although the two national ballet companies (The Royal Ballet and Birmingham Royal Ballet) are run by men, practically every other dance company in the UK is organised by a woman. It should cause disquiet that the situation in dance so often resembles an old-fashioned, traditional home, with the woman behind the scenes, nurturing and encouraging, equipping and being practical. It all falls into line with supposedly quaint ideas about women not wanting to put themselves first and having a terrific eye for detail (which is an essential attribute for any arts manager). This is less true in the USA and Europe, where there are more high-flying female choreographers and many companies or management agencies are run by men.

A dancer with many years experience recently observed:

> The trouble is the manager is often dumped with everything. They are always where the buck stops. The manager is left keeping the board, the dancers, the technical team, the composer, the sacked designer, the photographer, the driver and the venue's hysterical marketing assistant happy. I've been in situations where the manager has to cope with a smoke machine not working in a theatre 150 miles away from the office, because the artistic director and the technicians are not capable of taking constructive, speedy action. Or suddenly the manager is phoned from Tokyo because the artistic director has overslept, missed his flight and wants his office to sort it out. No wonder these people get fed up and burnt out!

Many managers do feel that the same old problems keep coming up and that they never get the chance to move on from doing the mundane tasks.

The most important characteristic is to be passionate about the artistic work you are managing. You have to be good friends with your artistic director: you have to trust each other. The essential qualities for dance managers are reliability, common sense, a facility with finance and juggling figures, plus an ability to speed through a number of detailed, relatively simple tasks very quickly. A manager needs to be practical and able to communicate effectively with an extraordinary range of people, from 'tortured composers' to immigration officials, from caretakers to TV executives. You have to be able to remember the names of a myriad of useful contacts, cope with conflicting, contradictory demands and sweet-talk your way through any number of tricky situations. You must have a strong sense of responsibility, but not to the point where it endlessly keeps you awake in the middle of the night writing lists. Inevitably, you must have a brilliant sense of humour. It also helps to be able to type and talk simultaneously.

Managers obviously gain practical experience on the job and all of us will have gone through 'baptisms of fire' and crawled painfully up steep learning curves. Some attributes are much harder to acquire: subtlety about when to pester the preoccupied artistic director, intuition about the delicacy of the creative process unfolding in the studio and, most importantly, the ability to give artists the maximum freedom in their work. Yet the rewards are numerous. What you get out of the job is a very exclusive thing: the closest relationship with the artists and the artistic process. You can usually get to laugh quite a bit, work the hours you decide, develop idiosyncratic and intricate filing systems, and choose where you want the office. Your artistic director can be the catalyst to a fabulous network of useful arts contacts worldwide.

Managing the product: distribution and audiences

Managing artists necessarily involves managing the artistic product and ensuring that the work reaches its audience. One of the key predicaments for the manager in England is booking a UK tour that makes any kind of sense in terms of geography and chronology. In return for particular amounts of public subsidy, funding bodies want 'accessibility' and prescribed numbers of dates. The pressure is on to come up with performances showing a nice geographical spread all over England. This presents serious difficulties as there is already a log jam of too many under-resourced dance companies (certainly the middle- and small-scale ones) chasing too few dates. There are few suitable theatres in terms of stage size, number of seats, technical equipment and ability to attract an audience for contemporary dance. Even more debilitating is the small number of venue managers and promoters knowledgeable about dance and enthusiastic about presenting it. With its technical demands and limited marketing resources, contemporary dance is considered a financial risk and something that audiences are nervous about. Most venues, therefore, offer short runs (usually one or two nights), which increases the pressure on dancers, technicians and managers. Generally, theatres are more interested in dance companies that can offer accessible, easy to sell work (such as flamenco and ballet). Venues also like well-organised education programmes and choreographers willing to teach a workshop to local dancers.

Barbara Matthews, manager of Cheek by Jowl (a successful touring theatre company) advises: 'don't make the promoter feel guilty'. It is hard, however, not to feel resentful when your calls are left unanswered and promotional videos are eventually sent back with a blank complimentary slip. When it comes to getting performance dates, all the energy and enthusiasm has to come from a desperately active dance manager. Managers anxious to achieve the funding body's quota of dates may end up agreeing to the company performing in a 6m x 6m space, with disastrous consequences. Unsuitable theatres can create nightmares for artistic directors, dancers and technicians, and leave the company's technical manager wondering about the effectiveness of Lottery capital money being spent on refurbishment. Theatres expect photographs, posters and leaflets in great quantity from companies, often before you even have a title, costumes or a team of dancers. UK performance fees bear little relation to overheads and related costs, so that a bedrock of public subsidy behind the operation is essential.

There are one or two honourable exceptions to the tradition of theatre managers who are drama, rather than dance, enthusiasts. England does possess one or two promoters who have done sterling work in building audiences and developing a context for more 'difficult' choreographers, whose work is perceived to be unintelligible to the general public. The level of communication, however, between UK promoters and dance managers is poor and they have much to find out about each other. At dance talkshops, Jodi Myers (Director of Performing Arts at the South Bank Centre in London) has repeatedly exhorted dance workers to consider metamorphosing into venue managers, as more dance experts are needed. The difficulty in the UK is that few venue managers are simply programmers, most have to deal with anything from pigeons in the ladies loos and worn carpet tiles, to keeping local councillors happy, making bar profits and balancing the finances.

The European welcome

In mainland Europe, venues are generally more welcoming. More theatre spaces are aesthetically suited, architecturally speaking, for dance. Specialist knowledge is more abundant, as is imaginative and ambitious programming. European promoters programme with sensitivity and there is an intellectual rationale to what they are doing: they are keen to travel to research their dance seasons; they talk intelligently about the art form; they follow the career paths of artists in the field and have artists' home phone numbers in their filofaxes; they have money to spend on commissions and co-productions; and they run big, high profile dance festivals. Most remarkably, they want you, they ring you, and they make a commitment. They will also be interested in what you are doing next year. For dance managers this is a huge bonus.

European promoters operate differently. They are not interested in thousands of expensive leaflets (the venue's season brochure is the main tool), nor education work, nor picking over technical overtime sheets to see how much they can run up your 'contra' bill for technical overtime or marketing costs. The fees charged relate rationally to the costs involved and the British Council (which supports and actively facilitates British work touring overseas) is often ready to contribute some support towards travel, accommodation and per diems. Dance companies are proving excellent ambassadors for Britain. The current Labour Government, elected by a landslide in May 1997, is keen to promote a new, fresh image of the UK overseas, and small dance companies at the cutting edge are doing this for relatively little cost. The other great morale boost is that audiences are usually so much bigger. Generally more broad-minded and culturally aware, they are willing to turn up and see an event they know nothing about. They are curious and take risks; maybe they trust the promoters! Some fascinating statistics could be quoted that compare audience numbers on the home turf with those overseas. Managers know that Shobana Jeyasingh sells out in Kassel, Germany and that Jonathan Burrows Group can get a keen audience of 700 people in Tallinn, Estonia, even if there is no suitable venue that will stage their work in Oxford or Cambridge.

The European model may not be directly transferable to the English context. It depends on different funding structures and, significantly, a more courageous attitude to art. England seems to be strong in areas such as education, training, and mounting successful musicals, but less comfortable with the cutting edge and 'art for art's sake'.

Managing the resources: funding bodies, finance and legal frameworks

Subtle, creative management of resources is essential to survival on the small- and middle-scale. A good tour is essential to keep the dancers working over a sustained period. It also makes the budget, which will be scrutinised by funders, board members and your accountant, look healthy in terms of earned income versus public subsidy. Running the budget is the most nerve-shredding aspect of the manager's job; it causes loss of sleep and grey hairs. Questions such as how much will the composer's publishers want, what balance should there be between the costs of design and distribution of posters, and whether the company should invest in hiring a van that will not break down halfway across Belgium, spring to mind. The budget is always discussed at length with the artistic director and at intervals with the board, but essentially it is your creative project and responsibility.

The struggle with limited resources is constant, even down to whether letters should go out first or second class. Flexibility must be built in: artists change their minds, the creative process takes unexpected turns and accidents happen. The beautiful, expensive costumes might tear in rehearsal and have to be repaired at great cost; you might need suddenly to find money for an osteopath to get one of the dancers back on stage; the designer might present a fantastic idea to the choreographer which costs 20 per cent more than the money allocated for the set; and the trust you sent a promotional pack off to might unexpectedly come up with £10000, while the £6000 worth of touring in South America might suddenly be cancelled. The unpredictable must be anticipated and funding officers are right to insist on contingencies being carefully husbanded.

Accountability to funding bodies is labour intensive and there is considerable paperwork involved. Artists who receive substantial amounts of money from the Arts Council of England and Regional Arts Boards have to submit quarterly updates and, for each financial year, audited accounts. Sometimes the cheques can be painfully slow to arrive and cashflow becomes a serious worry. There are annual reviews, appraisals, show reports about the artistic work and a host of letters and documents that keep filing trays full. It is often less time-consuming dealing with private trusts and foundations, as these tend to be less concerned with accountability. The crucial role the manager plays in brokering between the artists' ideas and the necessarily numerous sources of finance, is now the most time-consuming aspect of the job. Presenting artistic ideas and plans on application forms is just one of the ways in which the manager translates between the artist and the rest of the world.

In small offices the legal frameworks can be daunting. You can be breaking the law in blissful ignorance or a forgetful hurry. Finding a way around PAYE (Pay As You Earn income tax) and VAT (Value Added Tax) is mind-boggling, and VAT becomes unfathomable when overseas work is involved. Slick training courses give you a certain facility and familiarity with the paperwork, but reality is idiosyncratic. Instruction manuals will not give all the answers. This is one of the many occasions when you need to talk something through, in a concise and simple fashion, with one of your patient, supportive and more experienced dance administrator colleagues.

Money has to be ruthlessly controlled. Any artistic director with a tendency to buy expensive leather belts for the costumes on a whim, or to agree to a huge commission fee that is not in the budget, for an idolised lighting designer, needs to be kept on a short leash and without a cheque book. Managers cannot be secretive about budgets. When it comes to administrative, technical and artistic staff spending money, it is important to cultivate good teamwork, with communication, trust and respect.

Support systems

Boards of directors can provide objective views, fresh insights and encouragement. Quarterly board meetings are often useful milestones for the workers: an opportunity to reflect on what has been achieved, identify the major challenges and check the financial position. Board members can provide clear expertise and excellent practical suggestions, and the meetings are helpful forums for solving problems, offering new ways forward and building the team. Managers also need to talk to board members between meetings for advice, solace or information and to keep them up to date with developments.

Sometimes, however, it might appear that board members are amateur players in the arts, who waste time with pet theories and push irrelevant and vested interests, instead of letting the professionals get on with the job. The meetings might be quagmires of inappropriate philosophising with funding officers, who sit 'sphinx-like', taking notes. Board members can feel apprehensive about quizzing an exhausted manager. Many dance companies may not have boards or have only small, embryonic boards not yet in touch with the issues that matter. The friends invited to join may be clever and interesting people, but the meetings may not be useful for the workers. A strong chairman and influential board members can work wonders for a company, therefore the hunt for new, viable board members with the right range of skills and personal contacts is constant.

Your team: artists, technicians and the rest

However senior, experienced or eminent a manager is, at regular intervals he or she will lug boxes of publicity material across foyers and carry technical equipment through the rain. Dance managers are part of the team responsible for 'getting the show on the road' and that team increases in size in the run-up to a new production. The company's technical director is the manager's (and artistic director's) reliable ally. Managers must take on someone for this job whom they trust and respect. The technical director needs to tune in to what the artistic director wants to achieve in both a practical and aesthetic sense. In dance it is particularly important to engage someone who can realise the production values and quality of presentation the company is aiming for: for instance, can this person make sure the lino is flat and clean, and reproduce the lighting design in a converted corn exchange or tiny town hall? Communication should flow freely between the office and the rehearsal room or theatre (most likely running up a substantial bill for calls to mobile phones). The manager needs to tell the technical director how much he or she can spend under various budget headings. You might need to open accounts rapidly with obscure hire shops and check out the cost of building a special table that can withstand the fall and thump of human bodies crashing into it.

There will have to be give and take. The technical director has to be efficient about keeping track of paperwork and petty cash, and the manager needs to get cheques dispatched promptly. The manager should, if possible, be present at the theatre for the technical run or dress rehearsal. It is important to feel and behave as part of the team and this is one of the rewards of the job. Being at the theatre very early on the opening night, or the day before, means you can sit and gossip with the dancers and make sure the promoter knows your face. You can, of course, also irritate the theatre staff by checking up on the prominence and tastefulness of the front-of-house display, box office sales and the horrors of the guest and press lists for complimentary tickets! It is a good idea to set realistic levels of expectation with everyone: board members, dancers and the artistic director. Give them a clear idea of what you believe you can achieve in the time available and in the realities of the marketplace. Informal communication is also important and occasional dinners for the team should be organised. During the intense period of putting new work onto the stage and before the public, most of the axioms about working and staying friends with your artistic director should be applied with particular vigour: never spend more than 40 minutes with the artistic director on the phone (especially if one of you is at home); respect each other's time and supply of fax paper; and ask each other's advice freely, rather than assume an inability to deal with each other's specialist areas. Sometimes there is too much focus on the relationship with the artistic director, but this can be kept in perspective by maintaining close ties with the dancers and other collaborators.

Managers can make or break a company or a choreographer's career. They also need to be mindful of their own careers, continuing to be ambitious for themselves as well as the artists they enjoy working with. The job of the dance manager can be demanding, frustrating and lonely. They must be self-motivated but not egotistical, and adept at selling and marketing while demonstrating artistic sensibilities. Managers need to be good with time, money and people, and not averse to stuffing envelopes or helping with the ironing. Dance managers are experts in a multi-task workplace, and can experience gloriously unpredictable days in the office and on the road.

References

MacMillan, K. (1991) Introduction in Nijinsky, V. *The Diary of Vaslav Nijinsky,* London: Quartet.

Videography

Channel 4 (1997) *Just Dancing Around: William Forsythe.*

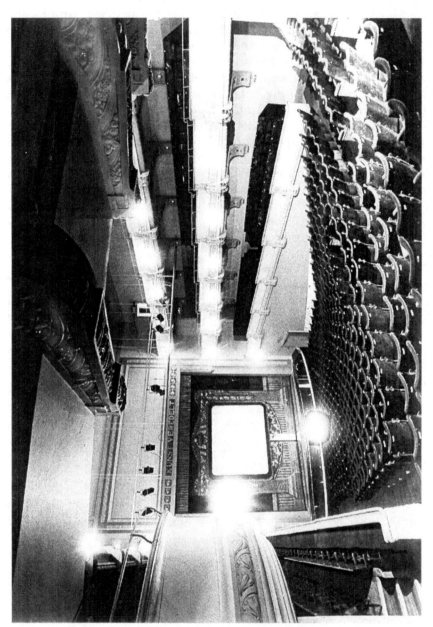

Vooruit Arts Centre, Belgium

4

Translating the Artist's Needs

Guy Cools

Dance as a professional performance art is relatively young in a Western cultural context. Although it has a much lengthier history as a social practice, in comparison to other art forms dance suffers from a number of structural problems, in both logistical and conceptual activity. Firstly, dance lacks an adequate language with which to write and reflect upon itself; and secondly, dance must deal with poor exposure due to less money and facilities for production, fewer venues for presentation and minimal attention in the media. This chapter sets out ways in which these difficulties can be rectified and how the artists can reclaim the time and space they need.

In order to gain the exposure an artist needs or deserves, s/he is dependent on numerous external factors and people, such as producers, promoters and critics. It is my personal conviction, however, that as an artist you can play an active part in organising your own exposure. It is your responsibility not only to create dance, but also to take decisions as to where, how and when your work will be produced and presented. The conditions surrounding both production and presentation are inherent characteristics of the work of art, especially for the performing arts. Drawing on my own experience as a producer and promoter, I shall discuss some of the potential problems for artists in organising their own artistic exposure and to suggest potential strategies to solve them.

The problem of time

Although dance has clearly managed to emancipate itself in the course of this century, its mechanisms of production and presentation are still very much dependent on the older and more well-established practice of theatre. Aside from the fact that, conceptually, many choreographers are closer to music composition or the visual arts, the practice of drama is still often the dominant production model. As a result choreographers are confined to rehearsal periods that are too short and compelled to create performances that must fill the traditional conventions of drama presentation; for instance, a performance must last at least one hour for it to be considered a full-evening's programme.

Nobody in their right mind would ask a young composer, however talented, to create a full-length opera as one of his or her first compositions. Within the contemporary dance scene, however, this is the rule rather than the exception. What is more, in many countries, the funding and touring mechanisms oblige young choreographers to do so once every year. Vincent comments:

> There is first and foremost an institutionalisation of the dance scene. For the companies this means that, once funded, they are obliged to tour their performances extensively... They are imprisoned in a more or less closed system they have to create one production every year to a standard format, from 55 minutes to 1 hour 10, that includes 6 or 7 dancers and costs about 1 million FF (£100,000). It is a product that corresponds to the demand of the market.[1]
>
> (1997, p.72)

Therefore the first area that must be defended is the right to spend more time on the creation of choreographic material. Unfortunately, in my own experience, it is very hard to demand this right from funding authorities, which, for most of the time, still use quantitative criteria. Although they may deny this, the majority of funding bodies are concerned with the number of productions or performances given by a company; and if they offer research grants, these are often limited to the period of training.[2]

If you look around, however, there are various ways in which you, the artist, can 'gain time'. For example, you can use workshop or teaching opportunities to experiment, without the pressure of having to produce a finished product; or by learning to segment the production process into different stages and units, you can avoid spending all your creative energy and ideas on one single production. At the start of your career, there is a tendency to focus too much on the production and presentation side, as you want to create and to perform as much as possible. Yet any mature artist would argue that, once you are successful, you will constantly be fighting against the pressures of performance, because the production and presentation schedules can easily drain your creative energy.[3]

What is true for the production side is also true for the presentation of contemporary dance. Venues dedicated mainly to dance programming, such as The Place Theatre in London or Théâtre de la Ville in Paris, are rare and only exist in major urban centres. In most venues, dance has to fight for its public recognition against a drama or concert audience, which has a much more established, and by nature more conservative, attitude towards an evening out.[4]

To escape the difficulties of creating a full-length performance, dance often looks to the mixed bill for the solution. Yet one has to be careful that the cure is not worse than the disease. To be able to present a varied and interesting mixed bill of the same choreographic signature demands an artistic maturity, and an extensive and well-developed organisational structure. Merce Cunningham and William Forsythe, for instance, both have a sizeable repertoire and a big enough company to present a multi-textured mixed bill. For the novice, a mixed bill often highlights various limitations and a one-dimensionality to the work. Meanwhile, the 'shared mixed bills' of most choreographic competitions or 'platforms for young choreographers' are often too diverse in style, and put the choreographers in strong competition for rehearsal space and set-up time. Nevertheless, an intelligently conceived and composed mixed bill remains the ideal solution to bring together the choreographer's naturally short format way of creating work and the public's expectancy of having a full evening's value for money. Therefore it is worthwhile being creative and spending considerable time on the preparation of a well-conceived mixed bill.

In practice, there are instances when the mixed bill format has been extremely successful. Traditionally it has been an ideal formula for a company to provide a platform for the talent within its own ranks and, importantly, to recognise the authorship of its dancers. It is also a way to confront the company with a different artistic practice from its own: for example, by inviting 'outside choreographers' to create a work for the company. In this instance, the unity of the programme is more or less guaranteed by the work having evolved from the fabric of a particular company. Two internationally successful companies who provide examples of this practice are Ballett Frankfurt (which, unfortunately, will never tour this type of mixed bill outside Frankfurt) and the Junior Batsheva Dance Company.

In order to introduce and promote contemporary dance to a new public, a funding body or independent organiser might commission and produce a carefully balanced mixed bill, by different choreographers or companies, that highlights the diversity and richness of the contemporary dance scene in a particular area. In Belgium, the French community successfully did just that with the programme *(E)motions* (1995). Three choreographers were each asked to create a new piece for a shared mixed bill which was to promote dance in cultural centres that had never before featured dance.

Finally, it is possible to experiment with the formula of dance concerts, bringing together choreographic and music performances based on the structure of a concert; the works are connected through a common, thematic link. For instance, using the 'piano' as a central theme, the Vooruit Arts Centre programmed a 'dance concert', which brought together dance and music from three distinct periods: the baroque era; Debussy's *Prelude a l'aprés-midi d'un faune* as a marker of modernity; and a contemporary composition by Walter Hus.

These are just some of the ways in which mixed bills have been successfully put into practice. The last example, however, raises a question about the relationship between the individual performances and the context of presentation. Although the presentation context can have a significant influence on the reception of the work, it is essential that concepts of presentation do not become more important than the art work itself. In relation to this, there are a few useful rules: the context has to be created around the individual performances as opposed to the other way round; the art works, rather than the promotional and presentational context, should reveal the underlying concepts of the event; and it is essential that the event should have an element of consistency through the various practitioners being at a similar stage of artistic development, rather than simply being part of the same event.

The problem of space

To say that space is one of the basic needs of a choreographer seems like stating the obvious. Yet I am constantly confronted in my daily practice as a dance promoter and producer with the urgent demand for 'more space'. This plea is made not only by young and emerging choreographers, but also by well-established artists. Since the contemporary dance scene is, by definition, an urban phenomenon, its major centres are also the major political and economic capitals such as London, Paris, New York, Berlin or Brussels, where the seeming luxury of choreographic space does not compete with the urgent demand for housing or office space.

Just as the need for time is as much about attention and attitude as it is about minutes and hours, the choreographer's need for space is not only a question of a number of square metres and a sprung floor. I once co-produced a choreographer whose work suffered from being over-serious and too intense, resulting in a 'dark' choreography. For the final rehearsal period, she was invited to work in the studio of one of the choreographic centres in the South of France where the windows of the studio opened out on to the Mediterranean. The result was a much brighter and lighter choreography. I realise this story may sound oversimplified, even stereotypical, but I have come across too many examples not to believe in the influence of the quality of the space on the final dance work. Indeed, as any architect can tell you, the use and design of space always reflects a particular mentality. Therefore what the artist needs first and foremost is a 'psychological space'.

The first condition of this psychological space is that the choreographer must be able to make it his or her own in order to really inhabit it. Shared studio space may be useful for giving classes or warm-up sessions, but it is completely useless in the production process. The creative energy of the artist cannot always be squeezed into a nine-to-five schedule. Therefore, schemes such as the SACD's[5] '1,500 hours for dance', which offers choreographers a limited number of hours of studio space, are completely out of touch with the real needs of the artist. Moreover, since membership is a primary condition to get this support, the real objective of this scheme is not to support the creative process, but to attract new members. In contrast successful production centres, such as the CNDC-Angers in France or the Klapstuk dance studio in Belgium, have always offered their artists in residence 24-hour, seven-day a week access to their studio space.

As to the desired design of the space, there is of course no single answer except that, in my experience, most artists like to work in a quiet, private studio space into which they can withdraw, but with lively and inspiring surroundings. They generally prefer a studio space with a 'view' and a lot of daylight, but that has the capacity to shut off the outside world if necessary. To prove my point, as I was writing this article, Alain Platel and Les Ballets C de la B were rehearsing a large-scale Bach project, involving more than 20 people, in our main studio for a period of six months. At one point, they had a night rehearsal from dusk until dawn. This not only created a different atmosphere and energy; it also put the dancers and choreographers in a position where they could take a different perspective on the material they had created so far. The studio, which is on the third floor with windows overlooking the street, was brightly decorated and lit for the occasion, while the entire rehearsal was shot by a film crew who had settled in a flat across the road.

What is true for the studio space is even more relevant for the performing space. In the German city theatre structure, and I suspect in most venues elsewhere, the dance programme is usually planned after the drama and music programmes. I know of one absurd case where this resulted in a well-established choreographer only gaining access to the venue on the morning of his world premiere. In Holland, meanwhile, most city theatres are so heavily programmed that artists are rarely allowed an extra 'get-in' day. Although such venues are undoubtedly well-equipped and have extremely professional technical staff who can manage the job in only one day, the programmers forget that a successful dance performance is not only a matter of technical efficiency. It depends on the artists having the time to adapt their work to the space, in order that it can be seen to the best effect.

Finally, it is not only a matter of access to theatre space, but also one of presenting dance in different settings. In order to emancipate dance further from the drama tradition, and to give full recognition to its own conceptual processes, it is important for the dance community to continue to invade and inhabit other public spaces, such as concert halls, rock venues, museums, art galleries, and even the street. This is the case with the recent hip-hop trend that has been artificially relocated to the stage, but only 'blossoms' in its original street context.

The problem of the dependency of the arts on economic and political objectives

Time and space are expensive, and the objectives of the people with the power to provide funding do not always coincide with the needs of the artist. When Antwerp was Cultural Capital of Europe in 1993, Luc Van den Brande, Minister-President of the Flemish Government, threatened to cut down the funding of this project because, according to him, the words 'Flanders' and 'Flemish' were not used sufficiently in the international promotion material. Two years later, and independently of the Ministry of Culture, he introduced his own cultural funding scheme. Dance companies, music ensembles, festivals, fashion designers and rock artists could get a substantial supplementary annual grant (up to £100000) if they promoted Flemish culture and nationalism abroad: 'Cultural Ambassadorship is an essential element of our foreign and cultural policy. Cultural Ambassadors are encouraged to develop their foreign contacts and activities in areas that are of interest to the Flemish Government.'[6] Since all major dance companies, such as Rosas (artistic director, Anne Teresa de Keersmaeker) and Ultima Vez (artistic director, Wim Vande-keybus), badly needed the money to support their international touring (particularly as the new fund replaced previous travel grants), the Belgian dance community was further drawn into the political and economic split of the country. The expression 'Belgian Dance Wave' was increasingly replaced by 'Flemish Dance Wave' in newspapers and other publications. Boxberger comments, 'Today, when the two regions (Flanders and Wallonie) are to a large extent independent and the possibility of complete separation is not excluded, the situation is more hard-line: in both communities there is increasing pressure on artists to visualise themselves as adherents of a single community and present themselves as such' (1997, p.25).

The relationship between the arts and the economic and political structures has always been ambivalent: from the feudal system of patronage, to the 'democratic' system of state funding, to sponsorship by private foundations and multinationals. The majority of funding schemes for the arts translate political and economic objectives into cultural projects. For instance, many of the funding schemes of the European Community, such as the Kaleidoscope or Interreg programmes, have as their prime objective the gentle eroding of traditional state borders; they insist on cross border co-operation among three or more countries of the community, which is one of the few, if not the only, well-defined criterion for funding. Cultural funding schemes are used to pave the way for political and economic integration. Similarly, private sponsorship schemes increasingly imitate the 'democratic' principles of state funding, using open application procedures with independent juries to designate their funds. In reality, this hides a well thought out media strategy offering the sponsor three times more media exposure: when the scheme is launched; when the jury announces its selection; and when the 'winners' promote their work. Significantly, the 'winners' are most often not young, emerging artists, but established practitioners who can offer the biggest return in terms of prestige and publicity. The result is a proliferation of cultural competitions and prizes, with the same handful of practitioners in competition for the funding each time. As an artist or company you can benefit from these schemes, but at the same time, you have to be keenly aware of the sponsor's objectives and the possible restrictions they put on artistic creation. More importantly, it is your responsibility to reverse this process and to find ways to 'translate' your needs into political and economic strategies; the verb 'translate' can indeed be taken literally, since it is often a matter of finding the appropriate language.

Years ago, before the Vooruit Arts Centre started to (co-) produce dance productions, I had to defend the long-term policy of investing in studio spaces, production facilities and budgets to our board of directors, most of whom were representatives from the political or economic sector. I had prepared a presentation on the artistic relevance of recent developments in the local dance community within a larger historical and geographical perspective. At the last moment I decided to change my line of argument radically, realising that, although most members of the board were art lovers and would certainly be interested in this overview, it would never be sufficient to convince them to invest substantial funding in this 'high risk' production policy. Instead I argued that, as an arts centre, we were a kind of artistic 'stockbroker' that administrated a 'portfolio' of artists. Certain shares, i.e. more established artists, are a sure investment, while others, i.e. young talent, have a higher risk potential. The quality of the portfolio, I insisted, did not merely consist of the individual values, but in the way the risks and possible benefits are spread and balanced over the different shares. Using language that was relevant, and readily understood by my audience, was effective; I did get my money to start this new production policy.

To some, this use of economic jargon might seem dangerous and a threat to artistic integrity and independence. Van Kerkhoven (1996, p.5) warns, 'the economic jargon is fast invading the language used on cultural matters and vocabulary is not an innocent thing'. Yet to deny that the arts are part of an economic system is as dangerous as sociologist Pierre Bourdieu (1980) and economist Hans Abbing (1992) have clearly illustrated in their writings. As Abbing argues:

> In the field of the arts, the use of economic language advances...The fact that the arts world is relatively reserved towards this, is quite obvious. It does not want to be reminded of its economic basis. At stake is the connection between the arts and unselfishness. The arts are related with 'higher' things and therefore altruistic...There seems to be a necessity to keep the arts world away from the world of economics and to deny the existence of the latter within its own ranks. The denial of economics in the arts world is a matter of utmost importance...In fact there is a big, financial interest involved in denying economics in the arts. Because of this denial, chances of financial success increase. It is because of the competition, the mutual conflicts and the exertion of the 'law of the jungle', as with anywhere else in the economy, that economics has to be denied in the arts.[8]
>
> (1992, pp.427–9)

To avoid the obvious traps of these double standards highlighted by Abbing, 'translation theory' offers a possible escape. Traditionally, translation theory defines a source language and a target language, and the translation process that converts the one into the other. More recent and sophisticated models[9] consider the relationship between source and target language as asymmetrical by definition. In other words, the languages are not only different in the way they are organised (linguistics) or in the way they encode the cultural and sociological context (semantics), but it is usually impossible to find a one-to-one correspondence between the two. As a result, the process of translation is highly complex and always deficient. It is mainly a process of strategic choices that are guided, on the one hand, by an analysis of the qualities of the source language and, on the other hand, by the specific functional purpose of the translation.

Applied to the relationship between the arts and the world of economy and politics, it means that when converting your own artistic needs (i.e. source) into political and economical strategies (i.e. target), you should always remain very conscious of the original qualities and demands of your work (i.e. the time and space it needs), the reasons why you have to

64

develop these strategies (i.e. to obtain the necessary funding) and the principles and criteria you derive from both in your 'translation process'. My own example, of the 'stockbroker' and 'portfolio' analogy, gives a good, although not completely innocent, application of this model. If you are creative, you too could come up with equally good examples for your own artistic practice.

At the beginning of the chapter I highlighted two key problems for dance. In response, I have addressed these issues from the perspective of the artist: how time and space can be most effectively used to benefit the creative demands of the artist; and the need to find an appropriate language to win the resources that dance deserves. Making progress in these areas is vital to the creative and economic future for dance and would, I believe, contribute to the maturing of the art form.

Notes

1. I realise this line of argument is more pertinent for continental Europe with its strong tradition of dance theatre reinforcing this. In the United States and Great Britain the modern and postmodern dance traditions have been able to deal with this problem in a much freer way. (Author's own translation from French.)
2. The increase and further development of private sponsorship schemes will perhaps provide more such opportunities since the need to invest substantially in research and development has been well-established and recognised in industry.
3. In relation to this Jonathan Burrows (dance artist) comments: 'Although you articulate the danger of forcing choreographers into theatrical models of working processes, my experience is that an equal problem is fixating on a role model from within the dance community itself. This can be just as stifling to somebody who doesn't fit the bill. The point is, there is no "right" way outside or inside the medium, there is only a "necessity" to work and the economic realities that that entails.'
4. It is no coincidence that the dance scene is organised around festivals rather than regular seasons. The festival format can be limiting for dance since it is often combined with other objectives, such as attracting an international audience of tourists as part of a general city marketing strategy.
5. SACD (Société des Auteurs et Compositeurs Dramatiques) is the main French organisation for the choreographer's copyrights.
6. From the brochure *Cultural Ambassadors of Flanders* (1997, p.20).
7. Author's own translation from Dutch.
8. Author's own translation from Dutch.
9. See Roman Jakobson (1959) who introduced the term 'artistic transmutation', extending the theory from the translation process between two verbal languages to any type of artistic creation using an existing artefact as a source.

References

Abbing, H. (1992) Art and Market Orientation: Exchange, Market and Unequal Opportunities, in *Boekmancahier* 14, pp.426–45.

Boxberger, E. (1997) Farewell to the Eighties, in *Ballet International*, November, pp.24–7.

Bourdieu, P. (1980) The Production of Belief: Contribution to an Economy of Symbolic Goods, in *Media, Culture and Society*, Vol. II, No. 3.

Jakobson, R (1959) On Linguistic Aspects of Translation in Brower, R. (ed.) *On Translation*, Massachusetts: Harvard University Press, pp.232–9.

van Kerkhoven, M. (1996) What are we Doing?, in *Etcetera*, Vol. XIV, No. 58, December, pp.3–5.

Vincent, G. (1997) Thinking about the programme in *Les Cahiers DAJEP: Art, Mode d'emploi. (II) Danse Contemporaine*, September No.30, pp.71–4.

MANAGING DANCE PRODUCTS

Introduction

Jeanette Siddall

Managing dance artists, as highlighted in the previous section, inevitably involves managing the work they create and produce. The two management processes are usually inseparable in practice, but they are distinguishable. The prime concern of the former is with ensuring that the conditions are conducive to the creation of dance work. This requires financial, human, physical, emotional and intellectual resources. Establishing the right to deploy such resources in the cause of dance is often directly related to the success of the resultant products. This section focuses on some of the issues that influence this success.

A key management challenge is to identify, establish and operate an appropriate organisational structure. This must provide the necessary legal and fiscal safeguards, while making a positive contribution to the success of the company, without constraining the creativity of the artists. Deborah Barnard explores the issue of company structure from the perspective of Ludus Dance which is a co-operative. She outlines the strategies that the company employs to ensure the structure works to serve its purpose, making the useful distinction between structure, leadership and management. While acknowledging the popular perception of the co-operative as being rooted in 1970s, as well-meaning but ineffectual, she argues that the underlying principles of worker involvement and empowerment are ahead of much current management practice. She goes on to challenge the traditional wisdom of the single vision, either of company director or artist, and describes the value of collaboration in meeting identified customer needs in terms of Ludus's artistic practice. The company seems to have succeeded in finding a form that fits its ethos. It could be argued that Ludus holds a unique agenda in which political and educational concerns figure as largely as artistic ones. This very uniqueness, together with the fact that the company has proved to be enduring, provides a useful model and a number of clear pointers for any small business, particularly one with a niche market.

Dance is predominantly an ephemeral and roving art form, existing in the moment that it is performed and roaming from place to place in constant search of audiences. As Anne Millman identifies, the total audience for dance in Britain is small and displays a relatively low level of frequency of attendance. The reasons for this are complex, and the extent to which any one characteristic is more significant than the others is not well understood. It is evident that marketing must be a key concern for dance managers and, rather than being focused solely on 'selling', marketing must be a constant theme running through every aspect of the management process.

Anne Millman argues the case for the centrality of marketing. She relates marketing effort to the stages of the life cycle of a product, identifying dance as a 'new' product. She goes beyond an analysis of the marketing challenge for dance to evaluate traditional methods and suggests some alternative ones. The customary marketing mix has evolved to serve the strategies employed by mixed-art form venues. Such methods are less than ideal for dance. Anne Millman argues that more personal approaches are needed to build partnerships between the producing and presenting organisations and through networking with the potential audience. She also calls for the greater use of 'new technologies' that can provide 'snapshots' of work that frequently defies description in words.

Dance managers often feel inclined to regard the promoter as a barrier; if only they could obtain performance bookings then the audience would follow. To an extent, public funding mechanisms promote this distrust with their emphasis on the number of performances as a measure of value for money. Possibly more significant is the extent to which supply exceeds demand; there are many more dance companies looking for performance dates than there are dates available. Linda Jasper explores dance presentation from the perspective of the promoter, and finds a somewhat surprising degree of commitment and enthusiasm for the art form. She focuses on a sample of venues in a specific area of the South East of England. The sample group consists of a mixture of size and type of venue, similar to that which can be found in other parts of the country. Starting with the artistic ambitions of the promoters, she examines the constraints imposed by the need to minimise financial risk, build audiences and justify the support of funders. Various strategies are employed by this group of promoters, including programming patterns, audience development initiatives and building relationships with companies.

The search for audiences for dance is, inevitably, a recurrent theme for all three writers. The significance of the audience goes beyond the income derived from ticket sales because it is a dynamic experience, rather than a concrete product, that is bought. The audience contributes to, and participates in, the experience, as anyone who has ever sat in the midst of an enthusiastic or enthralled audience can testify. Audiences can provide artists with motivation to rise to new heights of excellence in their creation and execution. They also provide a clear justification for public funds. This section provides examples of strategies that have proved effective in attracting these elusive, capricious and much sought after people.

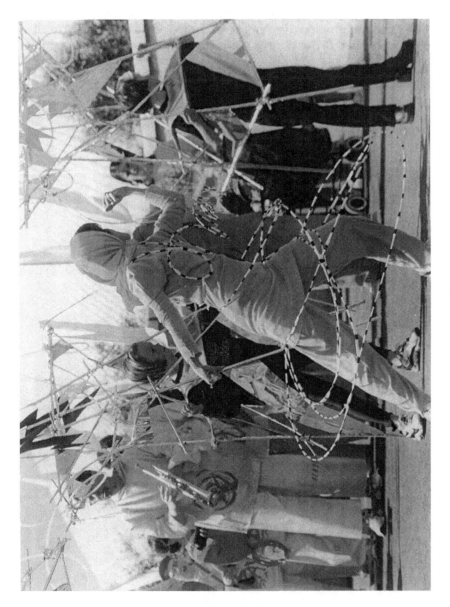

Ludus Dance 'Baybeat Parade' community project in Morecambe. Street carnival band encompassing music and dance, summer '97

5

Collective Management: A Step Ahead?

Deborah Barnard

Ludus Dance Agency is based in Lancaster in North West England. The philosophy and practice of the company, since its formation in 1975, has been to enable people of all ages, abilities and backgrounds to experience dance as a creative and life-enhancing force. Ludus believes that the arts can be a catalyst for positive social change operating within educational, recreational, creative, therapeutic and social contexts. Ludus seeks to realise its conviction by offering a public arts service which is effective, efficient and of a consistently high standard on all levels of company operation, from the delivery of artistic product through to the administration and organisation of activities. This chapter provides a case study on Ludus, and sets out to compare how it operates in comparison with current thinking within the commercial sector.

Introduction

Ludus is a co-operative. Declare this fact and the general response is a slight glazing over of the eyes, an air of nervousness or mild embarrassment. The perception of co-operatives remains rooted in the 1970s: well-meaning, but ineffective groups of individuals who spent the majority of their time in meetings, trying to come to a consensus, the results being very little action and no concrete decisions.

Over the years, there has been a line of well-meaning people who suggest that Ludus should 'become more businesslike', 'establish a board of directors' and 'develop a hierarchical system of management to direct the company into the twenty-first century'. Cynicism abounds and yet, ironically, many of the principles that underpin co-operatives are now wholeheartedly advocated by large corporations keen to maximise their competitive edge in an economic environment unsympathetic to 'average'. The human dynamic is again up for recognition.

The commercial sector is under constant survey. Consultants, philosophers, psychologists, sociologists and business 'gurus' have all contributed to the wealth of documentation and theory that primarily exists to support the quest for success, however that might be defined. Recent trends indicate the re-emergence of the 'customer', a motivation of the workforce, and the radical demise of 'the manager'. This is pointed out in a recent document, *Partnerships with People*, produced by the Department of Trade and Industry:

> There certainly has been a marked change in management attitudes and practices from those of the 1980s. This shift has come about from the understanding that it is the customer's needs and aspirations around which the organisation must focus. Also the realisation that the attitudes and commitment of all the employees have to be engaged in order to effectively meet those needs. Thus the best organisations manage rather than are managed.
>
> (DTI, 1997)

Periodically, throughout the ages, attention has turned to the need to motivate a workforce. A manager can work at a capacity of 100 per cent for 100 per cent of the time; this is effort wasted if not closely matched by colleagues or the workforce in general. Systems of reward, for example, promotion, bonuses and pay rises, have proved to be not only expensive, but are just not quite enough:

> You can buy a person's hand, but you can't buy his heart. His heart is where his enthusiasm, his loyalty is. You can buy his back, but you can't buy his brain. That's where his creativity is, his ingenuity, his resourcefulness.
>
> Covey (1994, p.58)

More fundamental human needs are beginning to be explored.

Anita Roddick, director of the Body Shop, spends 30 per cent of her working time talking to the Body Shop workforce. Roddick delivers lectures to her staff on the values that underpin the business; she engenders a sense of mission and passion about the work. In theory, we could question any Body Shop employee about the principles of the business, and they could explain, at length, the culture of their enterprise.[1] It is clear that the staff is a crucial asset. Peter Drucker (Koch and Godden, 1997) observes that the nineteenth-century employment attitude, 'people [employees] need us [employers] more than we need them', still prevails. He notes that this is no longer a valid maxim. Instead, words and phrases such as *empowerment, communication, sense of ownership, mission, passion, belief, pride, sense of personal and collective responsibility*, and *teamwork* are creeping in to the corporate vocabulary. Interestingly enough, co-operatives originated using this type of language:

> A co-operative is an autonomous association of persons united voluntarily to meet their common economic, social and cultural needs and aspirations through a jointly owned and democratically controlled enterprise
>
> (CWS, 1997, p.9)

THE LUDUS MODEL

Collective management

Ludus registered as a co-operative in the mid-1970s under the Industrial & Provident Societies Act (1965–75). The Board of Directors comprises every member of staff. After a period of twelve months, a new employee becomes a director of the company. All company members are legally and duty bound to participate in a system of collective management which operates in respect of all major issues concerning policy and practice.

Collective management does not mean every member of the company is required to make a decision all of the time:

> Co-operatives often confuse ownership and management. Because ownership is in common they think that management also has to be shared. Democracy, however, does not require that all who vote should also have the right to manage, or even demand a referendum on every decision. That way chaos lies.
>
> (Handy, 1994, p.162)

Democracy demands a climate of trust, mutual respect and a sense of common purpose. It demands a mentality that is concerned with the good of the whole rather than the individual, but recognises and respects that it is individuals who make up the whole.

Personal responsibility

The Ludus model is, surprisingly, comparable to the majority of arts organisations. The structure reflects the classic 'hierarchical' system with heads of departments, senior roles, a management group and a director. For the purposes of efficiency and effectiveness, the company voluntarily delegates authority and responsibility to particular posts, resulting in greater liability for the post holder. This could equate to the traditional notion of power, but, in the case of Ludus, the 'hierarchy' is powerless without the acceptance and trust of the company as a whole. The overall aim is to engender a personal sense of responsibility with regards to the management and artistic development of the company. Part of the induction procedure for staff involves a discussion surrounding the company ethos. Each company member has a personal responsibility to manage his or her own time and workload. If you are overworked, you first have to look to yourself to ask why. Subsequently, you have the authority to negotiate any change in your environment. Budgets are devolved and managed departmentally. More importantly, actual income and expenditure targets are set by department teams, and not imposed by the head of finance. Within this context, it is extremely difficult for a 'blame culture' to exist.

Not everyone is suited to such a way of working. In the past, members of staff have resisted the challenge of their own responsibility towards the company and have operated within an attitude of 'us and them'. Statements such as 'it's not my problem' and 'why should I...' are not accommodated easily within a structure that demands such a high degree of self-motivation and management. If people are used to working within strict frameworks it is often the case that, where a hierarchy does not exist, it will be created psychologically. This is a clear rejection of personal responsibility, either through indolence, lack of motivation or fear: with responsibility comes liability. Koch and Godden, in describing the future post-management corporation (less structured and more self-driven), acknowledge that 'to some people this freedom is genuinely liberating and stimulating; to others it is scary and paralysing' (1996, p.11).

Leadership

Ludus is not without leadership or management, but it does exist without managers and the traditional 'boss'. The director of the company does not orchestrate a group of people in order to realise his or her own single vision. The director is responsible for challenging, orchestrating and extracting the vision from within the organisation and ensuring the artistic direction is 'en route' to the company aspiration. It is an overview position that requires the ability to recognise and anticipate external climates and to ensure the compatibility of internal ambitions with those climates. At varying points, all members will be involved in a leadership role. The development of the education policy, training programmes, codes of conduct, equal opportunities, corporate design and so on, will be led by

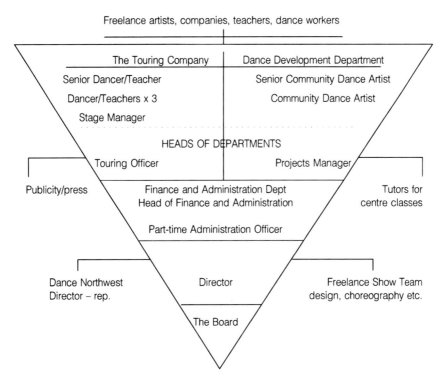

Figure 5.1 The inverted triangle

different individuals. As Covey has so aptly noted, 'efficient management without effective leadership is, as one person has phrased it, "like straightening deck chairs on the Titanic"' (1994, p.102).

The inverted triangle

It would be an interesting exercise for the dance industry in Britain to assess the layers of management and bureaucratic structures that theoretically exist to support the art form. Those structures could not exist without the artists. It is ironic therefore that the majority of dance practitioners exist within an insecure, freelance market. In contrast, the majority of full-time, secure and better paid positions are bureaucratic. It is an incredibly simple relationship; without an artistic product, there would be no managers, directors, development workers, administrators, consultants, advisors or funding officers.

In an attempt to redress the balance, Ludus developed a model of the 'Inverted Triangle' (see Figure 5.1), which seeks to acknowledge the significance of practitioners in relation to administrative staff. Basically, the artist works at the cutting edge, delivering the critical services direct to the 'customer'. It is the success of this layer that gives rise to the existence of the rest of the organisation. The aim, however, is to achieve a symbiotic relationship between practitioners and administrators. In terms of the Ludus co-operative, it is important to note that the bottom layer of the triangle, on which the whole organisation rests, comprises the board of directors, i.e. all members of the company.

The appraisal system

> According to White (1959), the 'master reinforcer' which keeps us motivated over long periods of time is the need to confirm our sense of personal competence; competence is defined as our capacity to deal effectively with the environment. It is intrinsically rewarding and satisfying to feel that we are capable human beings, to be able to understand, predict and control our world.
>
> (Gross, 1992, p.135)

As Gross has identified, we all need confirmation of our abilities. Ludus therefore employs an appraisal system that seeks to add to a process of confirmation and to develop an individual's capacity to be competent. Each member of staff undertakes an appraisal every 18 months or can request an appraisal at any time. The purposes of the appraisal are fourfold:

1. To establish a mutual understanding and satisfaction regarding working relationships and practice.
2. To provide a forum for discussion around any issues of mutual or individual concern.
3. To establish and negotiate plans of action necessary to relieve, rectify or develop and enhance work performance.
4. To provide a forum for positive reinforcement of an individual's competence.

In order for appraisals to fulfil a developmental potential, it is necessary to create a 'safe' environment and not one based on critical judgement from one group to an individual. To this end it becomes important that people are in control of their own assessment. Human nature often has it that we find criticism (no matter how constructive) more palatable if we have identified and 'own' the critique.

The appraisal is led by the appraisee with an appraisal team of two people. Each party has previously prepared a 'SWOT analysis'. Using an individual's job description as a guide, the SWOT looks at a person's Strengths and Weaknesses and future Opportunities and Threats. Other areas of consideration include staff relations, team skills and time and work management. The appraisee is also expected to prepare a short SWOT on the company as a whole.

STRENGTHS
WEAKNESSES
OPPORTUNITIES
THREATS

Figure 5.2 SWOT analysis

Ideally, one hopes for a concurrence of views. Ironically, people tend to be less inclined to identify their strengths than their weaknesses. The appraisal process often involves adding to a person's list of strengths, general agreement regarding weaknesses (with room for further exploration if necessary), and then a concentration on the 'opportunities' and 'threats' regarding personal development. A personal development plan is then identified.

Failing successfully

> The significant problems we face cannot be solved at the same level of thinking we were at when we created them.
>
> Einstein in Covey (1994, p.42)

As an organisation, Ludus needs to remain flexible in order to be able to respond actively to ever-increasing shifts in the arts economy. There will always be a sense of existing on a continual learning curve, which aids both the refinement and development of services and product. The company seeks to encourage an environment of continual learning; no one person (or the company as a whole) is presumed to be a 'finished piece of work'. Failure and problems need to be viewed as catalysts for change and improvement; risks need to be calculated and taken. This is not possible within a climate based on fear of failure and retribution. Therefore the aspiration, on most occasions, is to view failure as part of the job rather than the person; in effect, to 'fail successfully'. As Goleman notes:

> in terms of motivation, when people feel that their failures are due to

some unchangeable deficit in themselves, they lose hope and stop trying. The basic belief that leads to optimism, remember, is that setbacks or failures are due to circumstances that we can do something about to change them for the better.

(1995, p.153)

Artistic practice

Ludus shows are devised collaborately. The creative team comprises a choreographer, four dancer/teachers, a designer, stage manager, composer and director. There are clear agendas that the whole team needs to understand and satisfy. We have identified a clear customer base and the shows attempt to meet our customer needs. It is not always easy to find a choreographer who is prepared to work with such definite agendas and is willing to share the creative process with a team of people they themselves have not chosen. We aim to create a relationship of interdependence among the dancers, choreographer and director.

Once the show has been created, the dancers take on the responsibility of refinement and adjustment of the product throughout the tour. They manage their own training budget and devise their own programme for personal development. This can either be show-related or can concentrate on the advancement of performance and technical skills. The dancers will perform a show, on average, up to 60 times in a 14-month period. They will perform and work with up to 25 000 people during an average of 30 'residential week' blocks. A sense of product ownership becomes crucial in order to sustain artistic growth and to maintain the sense of journey and freshness in performance.

It would be fair to say that the working culture within Ludus translates clearly into the artistic work with young people and the community. The company recently returned from an educational tour of Australia; the observing dance practitioners dubbed our members 'scaffolders' as they provided a framework of skills and attitudes within which young people were able to explore their own creativity and create their own dance work.

Management

A management group that involves all heads of department and the director, meets for two hours on a weekly basis. Company members expect their head of department to represent them at this meeting. The group is entrusted to spearhead company developments both long- and short-term and to recommend the strategies necessary to implement a three-year business plan. The group also unites the various strands of

Ludus's operation and acts as a central communications point. It is not an exclusive domain; all company members are free to attend meetings either as observers or to present agenda items. It is worth noting at this point, that there is no job description within Ludus that is concerned solely with the management of the organisation. All members of staff, to varying degrees, directly interface with the customer base.

The minutes of the management group act as a crucial form of communication between company members. They are not only 'documentary', i.e. a reporting-back mechanism, but are 'active' in that they become an essential part of the decision-making process that is shared by all. Obviously, all company members are making decisions every day of their working life. When it comes to shifts, however, in either managerial or artistic policy, there are two main mechanisms: proposals via the management minutes or a full company meeting. As the dancer/teachers spend the majority of their time on tour, full company meetings occur quarterly at the most. The minutes are 'arterial' in their nature, and all company members are expected to give feedback where appropriate. Working parties are sometimes established to address specific areas of company policy or to progress certain projects. They exist for the duration of the exercise and are usually interdepartmental.

It is important to engender a culture where decision making is transparent and not the domain of the few. This philosophy extends to the development of the company as a whole, both in terms of vision and operation. The Department of Trade and Industry currently advocates the following:

> The whole organisation needs to know where it is going – what its goals are. However, if the vision is the product of one person's thinking, then it will have limited impact because employees will feel that it has been imposed on them and that they have not made a contribution to it. When the imagination of all people is captured, tremendous energy is created within the organisation
>
> (DTI, 1997, p.18)

Accountability and 'our customers'

At Ludus we are accountable to one another (the board), the customers and our key investors (public funding bodies). Last year, prompted by a course that a member of staff had attended at the Manchester Business School, Ludus undertook an exercise in customer identification. The aim was to look at how we could improve both services and product, in order to ensure we were meeting customer needs and achieving customer loyalty. Marketing the 'wrong' product or service usually results in a short-term, one-off customer contract:

> In one sense, economic progress and significant value creation flow from detecting or creating customer needs and then setting up ways of meeting them ... Being customer-centred in the right markets and with the right delivery systems leads to a virtuous circle that is difficult to break.
>
> (Koch and Godden, 1996, pp.5 & 31)

The exercise was not an easy one. Firstly, we discovered that our customer base was incredibly broad; secondly, we realised that we were neither effectively detecting, nor consciously creating, our customer needs; and thirdly, we found that our funding bodies are treated as customers in that we are encouraged to 'meet their needs'.

A single arts organisation may have several key funders in any given year; a Regional Arts Board, the Arts Council of England, local authorities both at district and county levels (often in more than one department), a sponsor, a foundation or trust, the National Lottery and so on. Arts organisations have become adept at rewording applications and reports in order to meet the variation of the funding systems' needs. Unfortunately, it is a time-consuming and confusing process that can ultimately detract from the most crucial investor: the general public. If we accept current business thinking regarding the necessity for customer focus, then to ignore the creation and meeting of customer needs, in theory, could result in the need for greater subsidy as customer demand falls. Currently, greater subsidy is not always a realistic option. Trying to satisfy too many funding agendas, combined with a lack of 'customer awareness' can lead to fragmented aims, limited vision and, ultimately, a weakened product and organisation as a whole.

The flaws

Ludus is a company limited by guarantee[2] with 'charitable' aims, but does not have charitable status. Unfortunately, co-operatives are not eligible for charitable status:

> A worker co-operative or anything like it cannot be registered with the Charity Commission who have a blanket ruling that no employee of a charity may serve on its management committee.
>
> (Cattell, 1994, p.34)

The biggest drawback of this ruling is that Ludus, unlike most arts organisations, is liable for corporation tax. Another downside is that some trusts will not award funding to organisations without charitable status. Despite this, we have always managed to demonstrate that we are a non-profit distributing co-operative, which has been enough to gain the support of many trusts and grant-giving bodies.

Postscript: is dance management ahead or behind?

Although by no means perfect, the working culture within Ludus compares well to current thinking within the commercial sector. The Ludus company ethos probably matches the 'post-management' corporation as identified by Koch and Godden:

> The post-management corporation will have authority and clear leadership, but the control will be based on internal motivation and results, rather than external supervision by the boss. People will do things because they believe in what the corporation is doing, and because there are no other roles available. People will not be supervised, though the results of their actions will be transparent to all colleagues.
>
> (1997, p.11)

It is probable that this way of working is not entirely unfamiliar to many arts organisations and companies. Ironically, over recent years the dance sector is appearing to run the risk of becoming a little too 'top-heavy' in terms of management, bureaucratic structures and layers of hierarchy. Koch and Godden (1997) believe one of the most significant hindrances to the economic success of large corporations is management. They argue that management is costly, adds complexity to both decision making and company structures, exists primarily to serve itself, and has little value in terms of direct dealings with the customer.

Co-operatives, which lack such burdensome hierarchies, are generally considered to be behind the times and incapable of survival in the cut-throat environment of late twentieth-century business. Yet Ludus has been in existence for 23 years. The fact that the company has survived for so long and now employs a team of twelve people is testament to the collective commitment and vision that has sustained the company in artistic climates unaccustomed to longevity.

Notes

1. This information came from a case study example, *Anita Roddick and the Body Shop and staff relations* at the Manchester Business School lecture as part of the Business Effectiveness Programme for Senior Managers. Devised for CWS, September/October 1997.
2. The personal liability of the directors of a Limited Company, in the event of the bankruptcy of that company, is limited to a maximum sum that will be declared in the company's governing document.

References

Cattell, C. (1994), *A Guide to Co-operative & Community Business Legal Structures*, Leeds: ICOM (Industrial Common Ownership Movement Ltd).

Covey, S.R (1994), *The Seven Habits of Highly Effective People*, London: Simon & Schuster.

CWS (1997), *Improving The Business for Tomorrow*, Manchester: CWS.

Department of Trade and Industry (1997), *Partnerships with People*, London: Admail 528.

Goleman, D. (1996), *Emotional Intelligence – Why it Can Matter More than IQ*, London: Bloomsbury.

Gross, R.D. (1992), *Psychology – The Science of Mind & Behaviour*, London: Hodder & Stoughton.

Handy, C. (1995), *The Empty Raincoat – Making Sense of the Future*, London: Arrow Books.

Kennedy, G. (1997) *Everything is Negotiable*, London: Arrow Books.

Koch, R. & Godden, I. (1997), *Managing Without Management*, London: Nicholas Brealey.

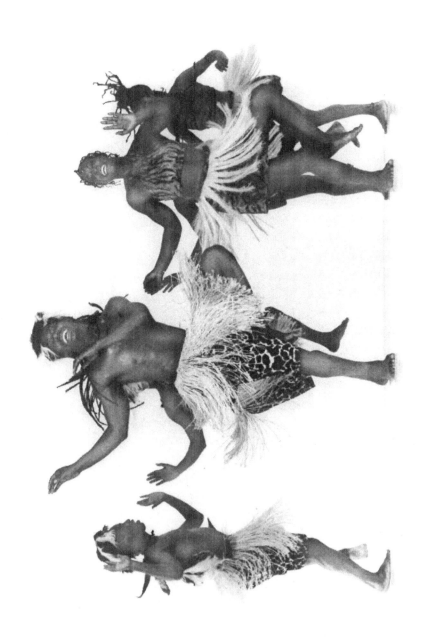

Adzido Pan African Dance Ensemble performing in 'Under African Skies'.

6

Marketing Dance

Anne Millman

To say that the core, regular audience for dance and ballet attendance in the UK is small is an understatement. Many more people are likely to choose a spontaneous evening out at the cinema, or plan an evening at home with a bottle of wine and a video, than to opt for a dance performance. In response, this chapter explores why the core dance audience is so comparatively small; the occasions when that particular trend is reversed; and how, in the future, dance companies might develop their audiences and profiles.

What is marketing?

In the 1980s many arts organisations began to incorporate the word 'marketing' into their lexicon for the first time. It was often used interchangeably with 'publicity' or 'promotion', and for some time few people understood exactly what marketing was. It was frequently equated with selling and, as such, had negative and threatening connotations for the artist. Now it is a concept that is increasingly well understood. Marketing is a process that runs throughout an organisation, from the early planning stages of a project right through to evaluation at the end of it.

> Marketing is the *management process* that makes the best use of an *organisation's resources* to *communicate* a *product proposition* to a *target market* in order to *achieve organisational objectives* and then *monitoring* how effectively this has been achieved.
>
> Verwey (1986)[1]

This definition underpins much of the thinking in this chapter, but before considering dance marketing further, Figure 6.1 defines some of the key terminology from this quote.

To add to the definition of marketing provided by Verwey, Figure 6.2 illustrates the overall marketing process and its various component parts, beginning and ending with evaluation and monitoring respectively.

• **MANAGEMENT PROCESS**	A continuous cycle of activity at the most senior level within the organisation
• **ORGANISATIONAL RESOURCES**	Human, financial, capital, technological
• **COMMUNICATION**	The most cost-effective ways of reaching the audience
• **PRODUCT PROPOSITION**	The whole experience, seen from the audience's point of view (the dance itself, combined with the facilities of the venue, and the overall social occasion)
• **TARGET MARKET**	Clearly identified clusters of people who stand to benefit from the experience
• **ORGANISATIONAL OBJECTIVES**	Artistic, financial, educational
• **MONITORING**	Evaluating success and informing future plans through an understanding of past successes and failures

Figure 6.1 Key marketing terms

If, as suggested, marketing has become more central to the arts in general, and to dance in particular, why does there seem to be a comparatively small audience for this particular art form?

Dance attendance in Great Britain

In 1995/96, four per cent of the adult population of Great Britain claimed to have attended a contemporary dance event.[2] Lagging behind jazz (6.2%), opera (6.4%) and ballet (6.6%), contemporary dance achieves the smallest slice of audiences for the live or visual arts. More critically, of the 1.8 million people who attended contemporary dance in 1995/96, only one in five went to a dance event more than once in a year. These low frequency rates mean that there is only a very small, regular, core audience: each marketing effort, therefore, has to reach out to first-time or infrequent attenders and cannot rely upon the cushion of a safe, core audience. Frequency rates for ballet are also fragile, with only four to six per cent of ballet attenders going at least once very three months and 12

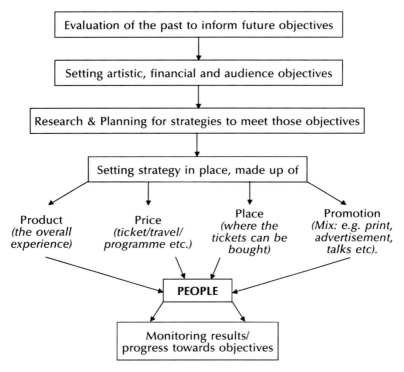

Figure 6.2 The overall marketing process
Source: Verwey

per cent going two or three times a year.

Perhaps because of the fragility of the audience base and perceived difficulties of attracting audiences, research into the profile of the dance audience has been extensive and consistent since the early 1980s. According to recent statistics,[3] the dominant characteristics of the core dance audience are:

- Women
- 25–44 year-olds
- Repeat visitors to dance events
- White/European
- Attenders at other arts events, particularly plays and art galleries
- People who studied to the age of 19 or over
- Social grades A and B (upper middle class/middle class).

With some exceptions (ballet audiences feature more people aged 45 and over than contemporary dance audiences),[4] this profile repeats itself in surveys of dance audiences across the spectrum of venues and dance types.[5]

There was a decline in the British dance audience from 4.1 per cent of the adult population in 1986/87 to 3.1 per cent five years later (1991/92). Ballet attendances fluctuated from a low of 5.7 per cent in 1986/87, to a high of 7.2 per cent in 1994/95, followed by a subsequent decline. The reasons for the loss of some 500000 contemporary dance attenders in only five years was never analysed. Crucially, the relationship between levels of provision and levels of attendance has never been assessed: in the mid-1980s numbers of performances increased, particularly in the small-scale contemporary sector, which could well have contributed to the increase in audiences. In crude terms, one of the reasons for a decline in audience numbers could be a proportionate decline in the number of seats for sale.

The position has since recovered somewhat (the British dance audience currently stands at four per cent of the population), but this still leaves the problematic question of why the audience for contemporary dance, and also for modern ballet, is relatively small. There are constant examples of unfilled capacity for dance across the spectrum, from African People's and South Asian dance, to contemporary and classical ballet. Supply is exceeding demand. Furthermore, the average ticket yield per dance attender[6] has only risen by 11 per cent in the past five years (all other art forms have risen upwards of 24 per cent). This suggests that high levels of discounting and/or only minimal rise in ticket prices has been necessary to maintain audience levels. As a result, cash capacity also suffers considerably.

Factors affecting audience size

The reasons why the audience for dance is comparatively small are complex. The following key points, which are discussed in detail below, indicate why audiences are so reluctant to attend dance performances:

- Newness of the work (i.e. unfamiliarity)
- 'Isolation' of the work
- Inability to explain the work
- Poor/inappropriate communication about the work
- Perceived and actual content of the work
- Venue.

While all of the live and visual arts are, to some extent, 'forced' upon the unsuspecting public, dance is arguably the most intractable. A theatre company may put on an annual pantomime or musical to cater for the tastes of those who prefer light entertainment; opera or classical music concerts can always fall back on old favourites; and a ballet company can combine the family-oriented *Giselles* and *Nutcrackers* with more demanding mixed programmes. Yet for the majority of dance, sizeable audiences are hard to come by.

New works

When it comes to marketing, firstly it is the very newness of dance that is its difficulty. It is easier to market older pieces because audiences have built up familiarity with the art form itself, the creator, the narrative, or the music: they trust the product, they know what to expect, and therefore do not fear spending their money on a ticket. Figure 6.3 illustrates the particular challenges of marketing any product that is new or young.

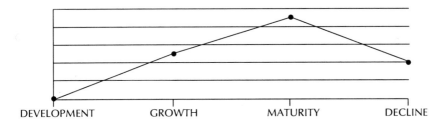

| DEVELOPMENT | GROWTH | MATURITY | DECLINE |

Figure 6.3 The product life cycle

During the initial period of a product's life, and indeed of a contemporary dance piece or new ballet, there is great emphasis upon research and development. The hope is that, with careful nurturing, it will grow and mature, and the rewards of attendance, income or critical acclaim will be high. In the later stages there will be a decline and, finally, it will disappear. Revivals of old and popular works can often be introduced to yield the rewards of the 'growth' and 'maturity' stages of the cycle, although it is important to identify when a revival might have reached the 'decline'.

The characteristics of products at different stages in this cycle are shown in Table 6.4.

This table shows that individual companies, or a whole art form, at the early stage of development will have minimal returns on investment, but will attract 'innovative' customers and have few competitors. The marketing response should be high levels of investment in order to expand the market; unfortunately, dance companies that are at the 'development' stage have very low levels of resources with which to expand the market, and this compounds the problem. The majority of

Table 6.4 Product life cycle: characteristics of products at different states

	Development	Growth	Maturity/ Saturation	Decline
Sales	Low	Fast growth	Slow	Decline
Profits	Negligible	Peak levels	Declining	Low
Cash flow	Negative	Moderate	High	Low
Customers	Innovative	Trend followers	Mass market	Laggards
Competitors	Few	Growing	Many	Declining
And the marketing response should be:				
Strategic focus	Expand market	Market penetration	Defend share	Productivity
Marketing expenditure	High	High, declining%	Falling	Low
Marketing emphasis	Product awareness	Brand preference	Brand loyalty	Selective
Distribution	Patchy	Intensive	Intensive	Selective
Price	High	Lower	Lowest	Rising
Product	Basic	Improved	Differentiated	Rationalised

companies at this level are on ad hoc, project funding; consequently, they are unable to plan ahead and they certainly find it hard to allocate financial or human resources to anything other than the production itself.

Isolation

Isolation is the second major difficulty for dance. Like an adolescent in a world of adults, it has difficulty in finding its voice and making its demands heard. Contemporary dance and modern ballet are, by definition, new and young, and are therefore less powerful than their long-established artistic counterparts. On the one hand, these products and their makers seem shy, almost frightened of their audiences, and on the other hand, they can be arrogant and audacious. They seek inclusion, but refuse to 'join the club'. They build links with literature, music and the visual arts, but can be notoriously precious when it comes to building relationships with audiences from the more 'popular' end of the same spectrum: audiences who enjoy ice-dance shows by artists such as Torville & Dean, or the large-scale spectacular revival of Irish dancing in *Riverdance* (1994), are possibly in the market for other dance entertainment.

Again, because of its newness, just as dance comes low on the advocacy agenda, so it can be isolated on the programming agenda: a mixed programme venue may include dance twice or three times a year, allowing little scope for audience consolidation and resulting in severe competition for those dates among suppliers. With the majority of arts attenders looking for a recognisable form and shape, familiarity, and something they can trust, all contemporary art forms face major barriers. In addition, like contemporary music or visual art, dance is, in marketing terminology, 'product led': it very rarely demurs to the needs and wants of the audience.

Understanding and communication

Difficulty with explaining the work, and communicating it to the potential audience, is another problem. Tensions lie between the spontaneity of the creative process and the need to pin down a clear message; between time imperatives for marketing (with deadlines often far in advance of rehearsal schedules) and the period in which the work is devised; between the inability or reluctance of the choreographer to explain 'what the piece is about' and the need to provide potential audiences with reassurances that they *will* understand, that it will not be boring, and that there will be familiar starting-points.

Recent research[7] suggests that people are inclined to stay away from dance events for the following reasons: there won't be a story; there won't be any words; the music, if there is any, will be modern, difficult or taped; there won't be much to see (e.g. in terms of the set), or perhaps only one dancer. Consequently, potential attenders fear that dance will be difficult to understand and boring. A further element that contributes to the difficulties of marketing dance is the nature of the venues in which it is presented. Essentially, the dance piece and the venue form two halves of a whole and it is vital that they are in harmony. In reality this is rarely the case. Subsidy agreements requiring companies to secure a specific number of dates, or to play at specifically designated venues on the touring circuit, can result in wholly unsuitable matchings of company to venue, and thereby of company to potential audiences. For all of these reasons, marketing and dance make uneasy bedfellows. Marketing has its sights set on the audience, and dance on the product. Contemporary dance and modern ballet may view marketing as a necessary evil, an essential link between itself and the audience: marketing can see dance as uncompromising and demanding, a difficult patient that needs careful nurturing. At root, there are many cases where there is a huge (and sometimes founded) fear that the marketing tail will wag the artistic dog: the rejoinder might be that a wagging tail is the sign of a happy dog!

Yet not all is negative. There are also many examples where marketing and dance make the compromises necessary to reach out to the audience without prejudicing the product itself: where marketing teaches dance about realism, and dance teaches marketing about vision; where there is an understanding that the product and the marketing function are inextricably linked; and where there is a mutual respect for an exclusive set of skills, and a sensitivity to the fact that it is possible to communicate clearly with an audience, without compromising the art form.

Some types of dance (and dance companies) are self-evidently more easy to communicate, and therefore to market, than others. In particular, those which include or deal with the following:

- Plot, story, or narrative components
- Strong visual elements, such as costume and set
- Sex or gender
- Specific themes or cultural identities.

The audience's desire for plot and story, and narratives that are predictable, is one of the major appeals of traditional full-length ballets. Research also suggests that a narrative element in a shorter contemporary dance piece or modern ballet can be a particular attraction. Likewise, the assurance of costumes and sets, the spectacular elements of theatre-going, is important. Individual pieces by British contemporary companies Rambert Dance Company and London Contemporary Dance Theatre[8] in the 1980s proved that 'sex' can sell dance (for example, the all-male *Troy Game* (1974) choreographed by Robert North). A focus upon gender issues also sells, as exemplified by British companies such as the all-male Featherstonehaughs and all-female Cholmondeleys. Meanwhile, dances that focus upon specific political issues like DV8 Physical Theatre, whose work often centres on sexual politics and gay issues, or companies that have a strong cultural identity, such as the contemporary African Caribbean company, Irie, or solo Kathak dancer Nahid Siddiqui can find their way more easily to specific interest groups and niche markets.

Venue

There are also ways of broadening the audience, which demonstrate the importance of the relationship between the dance and the venue. The product, from the audience's point of view, is the combination of both the artistic show on the stage and the experience offered by the venue.

94

Consequently, there are a number of ways of developing dance audiences. One approach is to present dance in a theatre not traditionally associated with dance: for example, Adventure in Motion Pictures (AMP) performed *Cinderella* (1997) at the Piccadilly Theatre in London's West End; and in the late-1980s, Rambert Dance Company did a season at the Big Top tent in Battersea Park. This approach enables audiences to come across dance, perhaps for the first time, in an environment that is more familiar and perceived as less specialist than the Sadler's Wells Theatre, for example.

A second strategy is to present work that is appropriate to a venue with a radically different catchment: for example, Britain's largest African dance company, Adzido Pan African Dance Ensemble performed *Thand Abantwana* (1997) at the Hackney Empire Theatre (a predominantly drama/comedy house rather than a dance house), where a large proportion of the local population is African Caribbean. The profile of the audience for these performances was predominantly African Caribbean,[9] and quite unlike that achieved by the company at traditional dance venues. The overall experience provided by the venue was more flexible and relaxed, with drinks taken into the auditorium and African Caribbean catering.

A third method is to present radically different work in a traditional venue: for example, Birmingham Royal Ballet's *Edward II* (1997) at the traditional, proscenium Hippodrome Theatre in Birmingham not only represented a departure in the company's repertoire, but also enabled them to attract a substantially younger audience. All of these examples show how major changes to the product itself (whether this be the dance piece, the venue, or a combination of the two) can result in changes to the audience profile and increases in audience size. Most importantly, throughout all of this, is the ability of the choreographer to see the experience from the point of view of the audience, whether that audience is broad or narrow, in order to provide a satisfactory experience. This is summed up by the comments of one arts journalist reviewing AMP's *Cinderella* at the Piccadilly Theatre:

> Perhaps, though, there is more to it than location. AMP has lessons for both contemporary dance (it always ensures there is a narrative to its works to help the audience) and classical ballet. Bourne is very much director as well as choreographer, whereas the role of director is curiously lacking in so much ballet...And then there is the marketing. Katharine Dore who co-runs AMP has concentrated her marketing on a database of theatre- and cinema-goers and not the traditional ballet audience.
>
> Lister (1997)

The dances and dance companies that are most difficult to market are those without any of the above elements, those that defy description and explanation, and those that cross intellectual boundaries. Examples in the United Kingdom include the South Asian choreographer Shobana Jeyasingh, who combines classical Indian and contemporary techniques; or Siobhan Davies, whose work, as one reviewer said, 'needs no narrative content: all you have to do is look, listen and marvel.'[10] That is not to say that it is impossible for this work to find an audience (Jeyasingh and Davies have both had their work performed in venues such as the Queen Elizabeth Hall in London), but there is a need for realism about the extent of their audience. This is where it is important to see marketing not merely as a tool for achieving large numbers (of people and pounds), but as a function that can deliver an appropriate, quality audience to a quality product. This is because, in classic marketing terms, such companies are in the most difficult position of all: promoting largely untried product to a largely untried audience.

This is most clearly illustrated by the matrix in Figure 6.5 which is used to demonstrate the different choices organisations have with regard to product or market consolidation and development. Box 1 is the easiest to achieve, followed by boxes 2 and 3. Box 4, at the bottom right hand corner, however, is very risky: an unfamiliar product being promoted to an unfamiliar market, with the net result that there is little to connect the two. Yet this is the corner that contemporary dance companies often find themselves in.

	EXISTING PRODUCTS	NEW PRODUCTS
EXISTING MARKETS	1 Market penetration	3 Product development
NEW MARKETS	2 Market development	4 Diversification

Figure 6.5 Product choices
Ansoff (1968)[11]

Again, the relationship with the presenting venue is vital. New work tends to succeed in venues where there is a consistent track-record of dance promotion (for instance, The Place Theatre and the Queen Elizabeth Hall in London), and which attract the dance-literate audience.

Stepping back and viewing the overall picture, it seems that while the dance forms themselves are constantly developing and evolving, the ways in which dance is promoted have stood still. The age-old mix of A3 posters, a review in a local newspaper, an A5 leaflet that causes an immense amount of grief to prepare, and possibly a radio interview is still often the main diet, particularly for the smaller companies. Furthermore, the venues to which they tour still demand this mix. Even for the larger organisations it is clear that this formula requires revision. There are frequent cases where too much money is being spent on general promotional activities, rather than cost-effective and imaginative targeting of specific audiences. Throwing money at the problem will not solve it: new ways of thinking will go a long way to improving the situation.

New marketing strategies

If the spare capacity in dance audiences is to be filled, some alternative approaches need to be called for: these revolve around partnerships, people and technology.

Partnerships

These would not traditionally come under the heading of promotion. The creation of long-term partnerships with appropriate promoters, may include traditional theatres and festivals, or possibly art galleries and non-traditional spaces. Those partnerships require two-way agreements of objectives; two-way strategies to expand the audience; and mutual levels of investment. Likewise, new ways of working will be to forge partnerships with those that intersect with the aspirations or lifestyles of the targeted audience. These industries may be fashion, retailing, publishing, media and technology. The proposition will not rest so much on the traditional sponsorship approach, but more upon a two-way package of benefits.

The London International Festival of Theatre (LIFT) has pioneered the concept of this two-way relationship between business and the arts and, most importantly, between the business person and the artist. Business has much to learn from the creative artist's ways of working. For dancers and choreographers the opportunities are clear: dancers can go into the workplace of a publishing house, advertising agency or broadcasting organisation, for example, and conduct workshops with the workforce on an ongoing basis. Choreographers have much to teach about creative ways of working with a team.

People

The second of these marketing strategies is the 'personal approach'. It has long been true that person-to-person marketing through mechanisms such as networking, talks or mentoring has a far greater long-term impact than paper-to-person marketing. For more difficult products such as dance, this is an area for exploration. Many small-scale companies would do well to dispense with their A3 posters and A5 leaflets and instead devise a more personal approach. Examples would include talking to existing dance attenders and asking them to mentor first-time attenders before, during and after a dance performance. Another approach would be to learn lessons from networking methods used by Asian and African Caribbean companies, which employ individuals within communities to spread the word (and the tickets) 'on the street'.

Technology

The third approach, and the one with the widest potential, is the benefits that dance will enjoy from developments in technology, particularly the Internet, videoconferencing, video news releases and so on. At the time of writing there are hundreds of dance companies linked together on the 'Dance Links' index, compiled by a dance videographer, on the World Wide Web (WWW). Unfortunately the majority are only using the Web to reproduce written information, such as listings, and therefore only employ the facility to produce glorified leaflets. There are, however, technological opportunities to address many of the problems identified earlier in this chapter. These include featuring short snapshots of work in progress, so that the potential promoter or audience member can view the work in advance: for the first time, it is possible to 'demonstrate' what the promoter will purchase and the audience will enjoy, and to overcome the barriers of attempting to explain the work through the written word. Choreographers and dancers will be able to talk with prospective customers directly, answer questions, and guide people's understanding and enjoyment of their work: they will be able to forge a more personal relationship with a wide range of constituents.

There are vast opportunities for sharing websites with composers, visual artists and other makers, and thus to access wider markets and make more lateral links. Merchandising opportunities also exist, either through self-promotion or through arrangements with compact disc shops and publishing houses who are selling their products over the Internet. And, finally, direct selling operations will enable smaller companies to target specialist, niche interest markets, much more cost effectively than they can through existing systems.

The scope that the technological revolution offers is enormous both in artistic terms and in promotional terms. Most importantly, technology offers choreographers and performers the chance to become part of a wider community, without posing a threat to their creativity or autonomy. It also provides opportunities to broaden the profile of the audience for the work; to overcome the barriers of newness and isolation, by joining a wider community and communicating more directly with potential audiences; to offset the requirement to explain the work in words; to overcome misconceptions about the work; to communicate its values directly; and to forge links with a wider range of third parties. It is perhaps the technological media that will offer most scope for the future of dance marketing.

The Technical Revolution and its Benefits for Dance

- Broadens the profile of the audience

- Enables more direct communication
  - to explain the meaning of the work
  - to overcome misconceptions
  - to break down the barriers of 'newness' and isolation

- Forges links with a wider range of third parties, including sponsors and promoters

---

Notes

1. Peter Verwey is Senior Marketing Officer for the Arts Council of England.
2. Source for national data: *Target Group Index* conducted by the British Market Research Bureau, 1995/96, + trends analysis 1987–1996.
3. Sources: *Target Group Index* as above; *Contemporary Dance Audience Survey* by AMS Marketing Services for the Arts Council of England, July 1994.
4. *Target Group Index* 1995/96.
5. For example, see *Developing Audiences for African & Caribbean Dance/Quantitative Research Findings*, June 1994, McCann Matthews Millman Limited for the Arts Council of England.
6. This is the average amount paid by each person attending. Source: Theatrical Management Association, *Prompt*, 1997.
7. Source: Since 1985 the author of this chapter has undertaken a wide variety of attitudinal research studies into the attractions and barriers of dance. These include studies on behalf of the Arts Council of England; Birmingham Royal Ballet; Shobana Jeyasingh Dance Company; Rambert Dance Company; and for promoters ranging from small-scale arts centres to large-scale touring houses.
8. Ballet Rambert changed its name to Rambert Dance Company in the late-1980s in order to reflect its mission more accurately; London Contemporary Dance Theatre was disbanded in 1994.
9. Adzido Pan African Dance Ensemble/Hackney Empire audience survey, March 1997.
10. *The Observer* as quoted on Siobhan Davies's publicity material.
11. Ansoff, I. (1968) *Corporate Strategy*, Harmondsworth: Penguin.

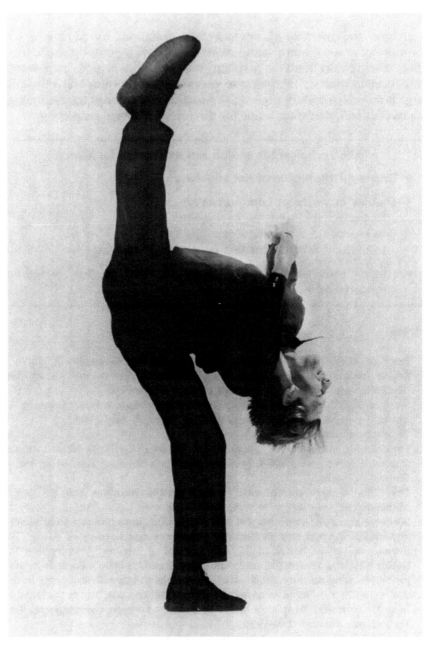

Photo: Chris Nash
V-Tol Dance Company...*and nothing but the truth*...
Dancer: James Hewison

7

The Venue Perspective

Linda Jasper

Introduction

Almost all professional dance companies tour and yet there is only one established venue in the UK dedicated to dance: The Place Theatre, London. Other theatres present dance alongside a variety of art forms, cultural events and general entertainment. Dance is, therefore, highly dependent on the venue manager for the context and the environment in which it meets its audience. This chapter explores, from the perspective of the venue manager, the key factors that influence that environment, highlighting effective practice and suggesting some possible solutions to a number of common problems.

The research for the chapter was undertaken in 1997/8 in a range of venues within Surrey, Berkshire and West Sussex. Information was collected from the venues through interviews with each venue manager/ programmer, written reports, and data from computerised box-office systems. To support this local research, interviews were conducted with dance programmers with a different perspective: Val Bourne, international dance festival organiser and programmer of London and Woking Dance Umbrella; and Marie McClusky, Director of Swindon Dance, National Dance Agency. Hilary Carty, Dance Director of The Arts Council of England, gave an invaluable insight into national developments in dance, and a regional context was provided by Sian Prime, Dance and Combined Arts Officer for South East Arts.

The Venues

The six venues that form the focus of this study are as follows (see Figure 7.1):

- **University of Surrey, Guildford**
  Programmer: Linda Jasper (Development Coordinator)
  Funding: Department of Dance Studies, University of Surrey and South East Arts

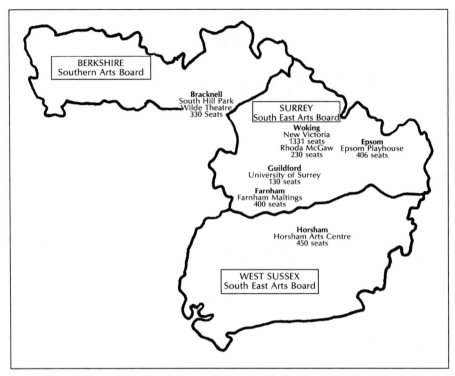

Figure 7.1 Venues used for research

Venue: A dance studio/theatre, managed by the Department of Dance Studies, that presents the work of choreographers working in contemporaneous dance forms.

- **Epsom Playhouse**
  Programmer: Trevor Mitchell (Manager)
  Funding: Epsom and Ewell Borough Council
  Venue: A purpose-built theatre, with studio space, that presents drama, film, music, comedy, light entertainment and dance.

- **Farnham Maltings**
  Programmer: Paul James (Director)
  Funding: Waverley Borough Council, Farnham Town Council and South East Arts
  Venue: An arts centre in a converted building with a focus on drama, music, participation, visual arts and crafts, bands, concerts, entertainment events and dance.

- **Horsham Arts Centre**
  Programmer: Kevin Parker (Manager)
  Funding: Horsham District Council
  Venue: A multi-purpose theatre and cinema, in an adapted 1930s cinema, managed by Horsham District Council. The programme includes drama, film, music, visual art, light entertainment and dance.

- **Wilde Theatre, South Hill Park Arts Centre, Bracknell**
  Programmer: Tim Brinkman (Director) Funding: Bracknell Forest District, Bracknell Town Council and Southern Arts
  Venue: A purpose-built theatre, adjacent to an historic mansion house, forming part of a large arts centre complex. The programme includes drama, film, music, comedy, light entertainment and dance.

- **New Victoria Theatre and Rhoda McGaw Theatre, Woking**
  Programmers: Robert Cogo-Fawcett (New Victoria Theatre) and David Vince (Arts Officer, Rhoda McGaw Theatre)
  Venues: Part of a purpose built entertainment and arts complex (run by Woking Turnstyle Limited); the New Victoria is a commercial theatre which presents large-scale musicals, concerts, opera, drama, light entertainment and dance; the Rhoda McGaw is subsidised and managed by the Woking Borough Council, through the arts officer, and presents musicals, drama, concerts and dance.
  Both venues are used for the biannual Woking Dance Umbrella Festival, an international festival subsidised and managed by Woking Borough Council. Programmer: Val Bourne (Director, Dance Umbrella, London)

Together these venues represent a variety of performance spaces such as can be found in many areas of the UK: they are a mix of purpose-built and adapted buildings of different sizes and economies. The research is, therefore, applicable to other dance venues and programmes.

ARTISTIC POLICY AND PROGRAMMERS' VIEWS

All the venue managers in this study are ambitious for their dance programmes. For example Trevor Mitchell wants to provide, 'a home for contemporary dance and new and up-and-coming choreographers'. He feels restricted, however, in implementing his artistic vision by its financial implications: 'we can't present anything ambitious or culturally enlightening.'

Kevin Parker considers Horsham is 'very much a ballet town'. He would like to work with, 'companies who are creating new work in ballet and contemporary dance and, in particular, regionally based contemporary dance companies'. He also feels restricted by finance, particularly the relationship between cost and box-office income. Robert Cogo-Fawcett adds:

> Delivering any progressive dance and/or audience development policy is difficult in a commercial context because the profit motive has to lead above any other consideration.

The venue managers are also clear about what makes a successful dance performance. Trevor Mitchell comments, 'it's a gut reaction, it has to be something that moves, that excites'; when he goes to see a performance he is 'watching the audience as much as the performers... looking for high quality print, materials and production values.'

Tim Brinkman programmes dance that has three distinct features:

> A genuine voice, [choreographers] who are expressing themselves clearly; a dynamic presentation [so] the quality and presentation of the work is exciting; accessibility, a dance company who can be approached by anybody.

He feels that, not surprisingly, it is difficult to find all three elements within one company's performance.

It is clear that artistic imperatives are not the only consideration for venue managers. They also need to take into account the financial implications of their ambitions and, perhaps even more significantly, the potential of their programme for attracting an audience. The constraints on the venue manager's construction of a dance programme are examined in more detail in the next section.

PROGRAMMING CONSTRAINTS

The venues

> Physical conditions of theatres affect the quality of the production.
> Robert Cogo-Fawcett

Venue managers are as aware of this fact as the artists. Dance needs a larger amount of stage space in relation to the auditorium than other performing arts; good sightlines are crucial to allow the audience to view dance that uses the whole of the stage, including areas close to the floor;

and sprung floors and large wing spaces are required to ensure the safety of the performer.

Companies (of all sizes) are becoming increasingly demanding in their technical requirements, which are often out of step with the venue's facilities. Extra time is needed for 'getting in' the production, for setting the technical aspects and for fitting the choreography into the space. Providing separate space for daily class and rehearsal can also be a problem for some venues, and the lighting of the moving body involves specialist knowledge, to which the venue's technical team need to be at least sympathetic.

All the venues examined in this study, apart from the Wilde and the New Victoria, were built without consideration of the specific requirements of dance; but Horsham and Epsom are particularly well suited to dance performance. The venue for which dance presents most difficulties is The Maltings. To quote Paul James, 'it is an under-technically resourced venue; it is a hall not a theatre.' Necessarily, his first criterion when booking dance relates to the technical limitations of the space and negotiating with the company – in his words, 'to make the right compromises.' He is often disappointed that the limitations of space have not been communicated to the touring company's technicians, who then complain about the facilities. He sees it as the responsibility of publicly-funded dance companies to tour widely, including to venues that might be technically limited for dance: 'ACE [Arts Council of England] touring policy is to get new and quality work into new areas.' This view is problematic for the artists: it may require compromising the presentation quality of their work and the safety of their dancers for the sake of a much-needed tour date.

This problem can be addressed from three perspectives:

1. companies could be encouraged to make work specially for difficult venues;
2. venue managers could become more aware of work that can be adapted to 'non-dance' spaces; and
3. it should be recognised that some venues are not equipped to present dance and should be discouraged from attempting to do so.

The availability of product

As a programmer I receive between three to five enquiries either by mail or telephone each week, to fill six or seven performance slots per year. Other managers also reported being inundated with requests from artists for bookings: there are certainly more artists looking for performances than can be accommodated at present. The New Victoria (Woking) is exceptional, only having the choice of one contemporary dance company and two or three ballet companies in the UK that operate at this scale. A further constraint is its proximity to London, which increases costs as some companies may not be subsidised to tour to a venue so close to the capital.

Despite the volume of available product, not all of it is of an appropriate quality: Val Bourne observes, 'artists at the small-scale will go up and down in quality; you can expect more consistency from an established artist.' A further concern is the relatively short length of contemporary dance performances, most of which, at under an hour, leave audiences feeling they have been short changed:

> Audiences in Woking expect to see a full evening's performance, not a programme lasting less than sixty minutes.
> Jenny Lowde (Woking Dance Festival Community
> Dance Coordinator)

Most dance companies start small and, in response to their expanding artistic visions, want to grow. To support this growth artists seek to improve the conditions for the presentation of their work, to provide better facilities for audiences, and to capitalise on a larger marketing resource and potential audience. In doing so, they frequently leave behind the small-scale venues that nurtured their early development. As the small-scale sector is the generator of most research and development work, there is a constant throughput of artists. For these reasons, the small-scale is particularly volatile, risky and unreliable.

The economic situation

A number of these issues could be overcome, or at least ameliorated, by a financial cushion. Kevin Parker suggests, 'If I could bring in a new company at no financial risk to the venue and the company, this would encourage me to take artistic risks'. Yet public funding is declining in total and fragmenting in terms of source, purpose and the conditions that accompany it. Val Bourne notes, 'All venues are now moving in effect to commercial status, which has been motivated by their funding position.'

This reflects a common perception across the country and is borne out in fact. Subsidy has been withdrawn or reduced from venues, due to the effects of many years of cutbacks in central government funding for the arts and Local Authorities, which has led all the venues (apart from the commercially run New Victoria), to refocus their artistic policies. This is a particular concern of Trevor Mitchell who has, over the years, used his subsidy from South East Arts to, 'act as a buffer to support work that makes a loss'. In April 1997 his subsidy for dance performances was withdrawn, and he has since reduced his dance programme which now includes more 'sellable' products. There is also the fear that funding will be cut further, especially as many of the Local Authority officers dealing with the venues are from sports rather than arts backgrounds.

Venue managers are cautious about applying for additional funding. Kevin Parker is not planning to seek Regional Arts Board project funding because 'it takes a lot of time to write the application and meet the requirements...it is not worth the money available'. He is also concerned about becoming too reliant on project funding, which can make the organisation vulnerable when it ends. Parker does, however, see larger amounts available from the Arts Council as worth applying for: audience development awards can range from £5000–£50000, and Lottery funding through the Arts 4 Everyone programme had a maximum figure of £500000.

Yet the Arts Council's particular focus on funding artists is called into question by Tim Brinkman: 'The Arts Council...only has a relationship with the company, rather than the venue or audience.' Kevin Parker also sees this emphasis on supporting professional artists as posing a threat to the venues:

> There is too much money put into new companies without supporting venues to put on the work...Venues are taking all the risk..there will be no venues if money is not available for them.

As funding declines, tensions become more apparent among artists, funding bodies and venues. If fewer companies are available it will not affect these venues greatly in the short term, but ultimately it will limit their choice. The Arts Council's practice of funding production in isolation from distribution is perhaps no longer tenable. Funding schemes that bring together companies and venues in joint projects or which link a company with a network of venues may indicate ways forward.

Other sources of income are becoming more important for venues, particularly in the areas of hire, catering, sponsorship; and the economics of the box office are becoming even more significant. At the same time, venues are reluctant to increase ticket prices: for example, at the Wilde, dance performance tickets have not even kept pace with inflation, having remained static from 1994 to 1997. Managers identify selling a ticket for an unknown event as the greatest obstacle to increasing audience numbers. In response, some are developing creative ticket deals. The Horsham Arts Centre promoted 'buy a ticket for the Vienna Ballet and get a free one for Richard Alston Dance Company'; as Kevin Parker noted, 'it persuades [the audience] to step across'. Such imaginative approaches, however, require subsidy. In order to implement cross-audience ticketing deals, Horsham and Farnham have both attracted Arts Council project funding for a three-year audience development project.

Trevor Mitchell suggests a way of making limited funding stretch further: 'I would like SEA [South East Arts] to give me a loan for £500 to underwrite a programme and if it does well then they get the money back.' This would allow managers to take risks, but it brings back memories of the 'guarantee against loss scheme', which eventually seemed to provide a disincentive to sell, as the guarantee covered the costs. It might be timely to reconsider how limited subsidy is used: old formats can perhaps be restyled to suit new conditions.

It appears likely that Regional Arts Boards will remain the main investors in artistic production, while Local Authorities contribute to the maintenance and management of the venues. There is an obvious gap: no subsidy for programming. Venues might be able to negotiate a better financial deal with the new unitary authorities, but it is too early to know whether they will have the political motivation and money to support the arts. The shifting of venues' funds from more profitable areas to subsidise other, less profitable aspects of the programme will increase, and managers will have to become ever more inventive if they are to have access to income from external sources.

Human resources

The perception of dance companies throughout the UK and other European countries is that dance programming is limited due to managers having a background predominantly in drama. There is a belief among some venue managers, echoed by dance companies, that there is generally 'little understanding of the needs of dance and the product; you don't get much commitment from venues' (Kevin Parker).

The level of understanding of dance is considered generally to be synonymous with its status in a venue's programme. The managers in this study, with the exception of Paul James (music and drama) and Linda Jasper (dance), are all from a drama background, but have a commitment to address any lack of dance knowledge through adopting various strategies. Most have acquired an understanding about dance through their experience in programming or in training their staff to become dance knowledgable. Some have employed consultants to develop marketing and education strategies for dance. Local Authorities have invested in Dance Development Officers, associated with South Hill Park Arts Centre, Horsham Arts Centre, and the Woking theatres. In Surrey, there has been a Dance Development Officer in post for nine years who works on related education projects with a range of venues. These posts provide participation programmes and actively link local people with professional artists performing in the venue. Paul James, like the other managers, sees an initiative of this sort as being necessary to find audiences for dance.

Marketing dance also needs special investment of staff time and resources. Pat Westwell remarked:

> More ground work and research needs to be done for contemporary dance; you have to be more innovative. The audience is a young market, therefore quite mobile; the challenges are different.

She compares this with selling traditional ballet: 'There is a certain pattern that you follow...the audience is much more easily defined and reachable.'

All art forms require a degree of special knowledge for effective promotion; however, less familiar dance forms require extra effort. Perhaps this, rather than the lack of dance specialism among managers themselves, prevents venues from presenting larger dance programmes.

The available audiences

Tim Brinkman emphasises the centrality of audiences to venues: 'the audience is the venue's product.' Attendance for ballet and contemporary dance is low, as a percentage of the population (see Chapter 6, Marketing Dance). Yet some dance can make money. At Epsom, for example, the profit from *Spirit of the Dance* in 1997 subsidised other areas of expenditure and Horsham's hire charges to Vienna Festival Ballet achieved a healthy excess of income over expenditure.

The most successful performances at the venues, in terms of audience returns, were ballet, flamenco, Irish and established contemporary dance companies, such as Richard Alston Dance Company and Rambert Dance Company. By far the least attractive events to audiences were medium- and small-sized contemporary dance companies. The New Victoria had more success than the smaller venues in promoting the same product, for example Richard Alston Dance Company and Jaleo Flamenco, indicating that factors other than the artistic product influence attracting an audience. The difficulty in selling small- and medium-sized contemporary dance companies' product threatens the continued programming of dance. Tim Brinkman comments, '[contemporary] dance cannot survive in our programme unless we can attract new attenders to the venue'. Ways in which to do this were suggested in Chapter 6.

Kevin Parker identified three elements that sell a performance: 'the name of the company; the title of the piece; and the names of the artists'.

In many cases, particularly in contemporary dance, all three will be unfamiliar. Even the more familiar form of ballet has its limitations, as Robert Cogo-Fawcett notes: 'There are only ten ballets that people will go to: only ten good titles.' This is evident in the difference between attendance at Horsham for *Swan Lake* (100%) and a new ballet, *Red Riding Hood* (23%). Only full-length traditional ballets remain a sure box-office hit. There is little evidence of an overlap between attenders of one art form and another. Robert Cogo-Fawcett stated: 'Audiences are relatively discreet; they do not cross over art events.' Neither does he feel able to attract totally new customers to ballet: 'we are seeking to develop taste in people who've got some experience of it rather than encouraging people to see it for the first time.'

An analysis of returns for 1996/7 from Epsom, Horsham, New Victoria and Wilde (venues that present a range of dance genres each year), points to the volatility of dance audiences ranging from 10 to 100 per cent of capacity (see Table 7.1).

Table 7.1 Samples of capacity for four venues analysed

EPSOM (406 seats) Average – 47%	%	HORSHAM (450 seats) Average – 44%	%
Hot Foot from Harlem	78	Vienna Festival Ballet (Swan Lake)	100
Richard Alston Dance Company	74	Vienna Festival Ballet (Giselle)	64
British Gas Ballet	71	Richard Alston Dance Company	54
Rhythms of Africa	48	Diversions	40
Shobana Jeyasingh	35	Cwni Ballet (Red Riding Hood)	23
Mark Baldwin	33	Jo Chavala	19
Dance Festival 1 & 3	30	Union Dance	10
RJC	29		
Dance Fest 2	25		
Cholmondeleys (site-specific)	100		

NEW VICTORIA THEATRE (1331 seats) Average – 77%	%	WILDE (330 seats) Average – 31%	%
Spirit of the Dance	100	Jaleo Flamenco	72
Northern Ballet Theatre	87	British Gas Ballet	69
Moscow City Ballet	97	Adzido African Dance	32
London City Ballet	75	Stung	23
Rambert Dance Company	70	V-Tol	21
Philippe Decouflé	65	Idée Fixe	19
Scottish Ballet	70	Momentary Fusion	17
Jaleo Flamenco	50	Candoco	15
		Green Candle	14

Dance forms attract different people, which clearly poses a marketing challenge for managers. However, their belief that:

> There are millions who would enjoy the work that we enjoy if they had the right opportunity; let's get out there and find them.
>
> Marchant (1996)

sustains the managers' enthusiasm for programming dance and continually devising creative marketing strategies.

PROGRAMMING PATTERNS

Given the challenges, the managers contained in this study are perhaps to be congratulated on the variety of their programmes. Overall there is a range of dance available to local populations in the form of African Peoples' dance, ballet, contemporary dance, flamenco, Irish folk, jazz/tap and South Asian dance. There were 54 professional dance companies presented in 1996/7 and 36 in 1997/8. The increase in the number of companies in 1997 is accounted for by the Woking Dance Umbrella Festival which was presented in that year. Table 7.2 presents an analysis of the different dance genres, and provides an overview of each venue's programme.

Table 7.2 Number of dance forms presented in each year expressed as a percentage of overall dance programmes for each venue

Venue	Year	No. of Co's	African Peoples	Ballet	Contemporary Dance	Flamenco	Irish	Jazz/ Tap	South Asian
Epsom Playhouse	1996/7	11	9	9	64	0	0	9	9
	1997/8	9	0	33	22	11	11	22	0
Farnham Maltings	1996/7	1	0	0	100	0	0	0	0
	1997/8	1	0	0	100	0	0	0	0
Horsham Arts Centre	1996/7	6	0	33	50	17	0	0	0
	1997/8	8	0	38	50	0	0	13	0
New Victoria	1996/7	8	0	50	25	12	12	0	0
	1997/8	6	0	33	33	0	33	0	0
Rhoda McGaw	1996/7	13	12	0	66	0	0	7	15
	1997/8	0	0	0	0	0	0	0	0
Wilde	1996/7	9	0	11	78	11	0	0	0
	1997/8	6	0	17	66	17	0	0	0
Surrey University	1996/7	6	0	0	100	0	0	0	0
	1997/8	6	0	0	83	0	0	0	17

The broadest programme is presented at Epsom, with Rhoda McGaw showing a similar range. The narrowest programming is at the University and Farnham, where their policies of presenting contemporary dance are evident. At Epsom and the Wilde, there was a reduction in the number of companies presented in 1997/8 and an increase at Horsham. Contemporary dance was significantly cut back at Epsom and reduced at the Wilde in 1997/8. Outside of a festival year, it appears that dance ceases in the Rhoda McGaw.

Hilary Carty stated that venues were:

> Experimenting with many different programming formats: one nighters, special relationships ... and in particular the emergence of the small-scale dance festival model where 4–5 companies might be performing over ten days to two weeks.

The festival format she felt worked well, a format that South Hill Park Arts Centre moved to in the autumn of 1998, with interval programming in other parts of year. The reasons for this were:

> To create a bigger weight for dance ... by grouping a programme together so that dance can find a platform, find increased investment from funders and sponsors. The dance attender can look at the collection of performances programmed and make choices about what they want to see: creating a critical mass of product and promotion to generate more audiences.
>
> Tim Brinkman

It will be interesting to see whether Tim Brinkman is right or whether expecting audiences to attend repeatedly within a short time period may be overly optimistic.

The Woking Dance Umbrella Festival has been enormously successful in attracting audiences from a large area and in promoting the town, as well as the venue. The festival is biannual, international in character and run by a separate organisation; representatives from each venue sit on the board to meet the heavy staffing demands of a festival. Although festivals can generate enormous interest, three of the venues have no plans to follow this pattern. For these venues the resources that it takes to organise and promote such an event perhaps outweigh the benefits.

Yet presenting dance companies at 'intervals' requires resources to be put into reaching audiences on a regular basis. Marie McClusky stated: 'Presenting odd shows is not working.' She targets events very closely and offers additional selling points; for example, Random Dance Company's latest performance was followed by a party with DJ and sound system.

The 'residency model' has been used over a number of years to develop audiences' understanding of dance through providing a longer term contact with artists, but there are costs associated with this model. It demands a greater investment of time and money from the venue and usually needs a dedicated worker to manage it. To be worthwhile it has to serve other aims: either to fulfil the wider education/access policy of the venue or the brief of a dance development officer. No one programming model will be effective for all venues. Each uses formats depending on the factors governing its operations at any given time. Festivals with the right level of support can be extremely attractive to audiences, but they are costly. Residencies can build a knowledge of a particular artist's work, but again require financial and human resources. Site-specific work can provide a profile for the venue in a different and, sometimes, more public site, but involves careful management. Interval programming works very well for most of the venues, but they are aware that certain companies will need special attention if they are going to sell in this format.

General rules apply to all the venues: contemporary dance performances, that rely on school groups, are always programmed on weekday evenings, rather than weekends and school holidays; and ballets with family appeal are presented as Saturday matinée and evening performances, as well as in the week. The manager's vision is central to the planning and implementation of all of these models. Perhaps this experimentation with different programming formats is not only a means to attract audiences, but also a way to meet the managers' need to produce: programming is the creative medium of the manager. Appendix 1 highlights the benefits and disadvantages of different programming, all of which are, or have been, used by the venues in the study.

ADDRESSING THE ISSUES

Audience development

Bigger and better-informed audiences are key to sustaining and increasing the range and number of dance performances programmed by the venues in this study and, it may be assumed, across the country. Meanwhile, venue managers hope that increasingly well-informed audiences will be willing to take greater 'artistic risk' and, indeed, may even demand it. 'Audience development' is seen as the solution by all the managers, but what does this mean? The Arts Council of Great Britain described it as follows:

Audience development has at least three aspects; heightening the experience of viewing, reading, listening to the arts and media; increasing the numbers of people throughout society who have the opportunity to do this; and assisting the process of mutual understanding between maker or performer and receiver.

ACGB (1993, p.36)

This definition goes beyond the instrumental use of publicity tools to sell seats: it embraces educational and social, as well as artistic, objectives. Yet increasing the number of attenders is obviously very high on the agenda of managers. This begs the questions, 1) which audience development strategies do they use? and 2) how successful are they?

Education

Audience development strategies in dance have always involved potential audiences in physical participation. Through deepening their awareness of dance, it is expected that participants will then be actively encouraged to be spectators. The education policy at Horsham exemplifies this approach. It was implemented in 1993 and has included four contemporary dance companies. One model involves the company leading workshops in schools, based on themes from the repertoire; the company then returns to the schools nearer the performance date, and a showcase performance of the school's work is given on the day of the company performance. A joint workshop and performance ticket deal is available to all participants. The Richard Alston Dance Company has been used most consistently to fulfil this policy. Research tracking school groups attending through two consecutive years showed that 39 per cent of schools returned, 44 per cent of schools did not, and the remaining 17 per cent consisted of new schools (Brennan, 1997).

There are many reasons why schools cannot take up opportunities to engage in annual projects and therefore this model, although instrumental in increasing audience attendance and heightening the experience of the pupils engaged in a particular project, cannot guarantee a development of audiences over a period of time. At Horsham, the only point that can be proved is that there is an increase in numbers of young people attending individual performances associated with the projects. Kevin Parker reflected on this aspect of his policy: 'It is a perpetual problem; people attend as part of a group, you hope that the person returns as an individual.'

There are, however, other benefits as Parker witnessed at a performance of Richard Alston Dance Company:

[There were] kids in the audience screaming at the end of pieces, there is a sense of ownership through knowing the dancers and knowing the themes; it goes deeper than an immediate response; they've made contact and go away with a much deeper experience.

Paul James said he 'doesn't expect large audiences for contemporary dance' and therefore asks the question 'how can you add value to the performance?': he answers himself, 'the education work adds quality.'

Participation

The amateur dance performance programme at South Hill Park Arts Centre illustrates another audience development strategy. The theory is that watching community dance performances in support of a friend or family member encourages an interest in attending professional dance performances. Yet a study of audience returns for years 1993, 1994 and 1995 suggests this to be true for only 14 per cent of people. Sixty-eight per cent of attenders of amateur dance performances did not attend any other type of event at the venue, demonstrating that amateur dance performances create their own audiences, as is the case with amateur drama.

Participation in dance has a value in its own right: people who enjoy dancing do not necessarily want to watch it. Unfortunately, venues are pressured by both the financial risk of presenting professional artists' work and the pressing need to employ strategies to attract audiences. Yet they need to recognise and value other benefits of participation activities, particularly in reaching a broader section of the population. Participation strategies also promote venues as centres for dance, raising the dance profile of the venue, and sometimes generating income without requiring subsidy.

Developing relationships between artists and audiences

Most artists make work to meet their own needs. Some care more about audience response than others, but all would agree that performing to an audience reveals if the aims of the work are clear, enables the performers to develop their interpretation of the choreography and ultimately effects the development of the artists' work. Not surprisingly there is a different view of audiences between venue and artists. Pat Westwell recalls the comments of one choreographer: '[He] said to me he doesn't care about the size of the audiences, he just wants them to understand his piece.' Similarly, Tim Brinkman adds:

Audiences can be seen as a last link in the chain, we need to move to a model where the audience is at the centre of the process... your dance doesn't exist if no-one wants to watch it.

This latter statement is contentious and certainly some artists have argued for the right to be able to perform their work before no audience, if they wish (Brook, 1972). Yet, for most artists and all venues managers, performing to an audience is an essential part of the creative process. Tim Brinkman feels, as other managers do, that contemporary dance artists, after many years of being introspective and not particularly concerned about audiences, 'have broken out of a box, moving towards being more accessible to audiences'. This new willingness by artists to communicate with audiences could be a response to the harsh financial climate they are operating in, as much as any change in artistic visions: if they cannot attract audiences then venues may not book them. In order to assist the understanding between artist and audience, venue managers are building 'special relationships' with some companies.

Venue and artist relationships

Hilary Carty views special relationships as being a very positive step forward for venue managers and artists when building dance programmes:

Some of the best practice of dance programming in venues is where managers are pro-active in commissioning and developing a relationship with a dance company... managers are finding it more rewarding to enter in a longer term relationship with companies over two to four-year periods.

Describing what these relationships include, she identified 'co-commissioning and co-producing, offering a space, technical rehearsals, assisting in shaping a product'. These points emphasise the benefits of the relationship from the artists' perspective. Tim Brinkman described his expectations of the planned special relationship with V-Tol as, 'working together with the company to find an audience for their work and overcome the rigours of touring; venues are the agents to make it happen'. This appears to be a very altruistic response from a venue perspective. Tim Brinkman suggests the direct benefit for him: 'In the end, the purpose is to develop more audiences and sell more seats.' He believes a three-year commitment is needed and highlights practical advice for an effective relationship: 'Build on rapport and trust, talk in advance, plan early, represent needs of the audience in terms of pricing and promotional channels, commit to a company for a number of years.'

It is unclear whether a larger audience follows this kind of relationship. It does, however, provide opportunities for a long-term engagement by artists with a particular venue, its staff and its community, and for a shared experience of art.

Product development

Cogo-Fawcett comments that, from a drama perspective, 'Audience development should be a product-led initiative; not a marketing one.' This is less of a concern for dance as many artists are in a constant research and development mode.

The expectations of the artists, funding bodies and venue managers, that a new work will be toured each year, demands constant engagement with creating new work to the possible detriment of consistency of quality in the product and thereby audience development. Tim Brinkman said: 'The problem with dance, as well as some theatre productions, is that they both suffer from the "make and break cycle", chucking away the best work.' He felt that building up a repertoire of a company's best works would serve the aims of audience development more effectively and that companies could become better known by returning to the venue twice in a particular year. Yet this is problematic in that the company would have to make new work, as well as building up a repertoire of 'best works'. The expectations of the venues could be seen as at odds with the research and development nature of the dance form. For most of the venues, contemporary dance remains project-based, and repertory work will be found in other dance forms, such as ballet and flamenco.

Direct marketing

As computerised box-office packages have been acquired by venues, they have the capacity to distinguish, categorise and abstract information on their customers with increasing sophistication. This has led to a more accurate targeting of potential customers across various dance genres. It has become the most important tool in audience development and marketing. The venues use computer box-office software packages that identify each individual customer by name, postcode, attendance record, booking patterns, and the effectiveness of the venue's publicity on the customer's attendance. The venues also use Arts Council 'site reports', which reveal clusters of attenders of specific art forms in different areas of the country.

Trevor Mitchell has used his audience database to assist incremental programming over a number of years in order to increase audiences for dance. In 1985 he presented the Brazilian Dance Theatre, which attracted

65 per cent attendance and all the audience addresses were recorded. Another large-scale dance event was then programmed which attracted the first attenders, as well as their friends. From this initial investment in high-profile company performances, audiences were tested on different products so that they eventually could be categorised by dance interest. Through categorisation, Mitchell encourages audiences to cross over to other dance genres. He sees incremental programming as a method of 'encouraging audiences to try something new.'

'Database returns' also identify core venue audiences, as well as core art form audiences: venue loyalty is a reality, and people tend to return to a theatre they are familiar with. Tim Brinkman comments,

> Audience experience is the whole thing, not just the dance; easy travelling to the venue, safe car parking, comfortable seats, good sight lines, prompt bar service are a part of the artistic experience. Artists need to trust the venue to be able to deliver the total package.

Venue loyalty is engendered by trust; the loyal audience trusts the programmer's choice, as well as the venue's services.

Generating 'word of mouth' communication is effective because it is based on trust. At the New Victoria, part-time 'District Publicity Assistants' attend monthly meetings where the future programme is explained to them and their work is co-ordinated. Dance company managers are invited to give presentations, including video extracts, and the assistants then go out 'armed with information and sell it to the public at a grass roots level' (Pat Westwell).

BUILDING ON SUCCESS

Tim Brinkman, when evaluating Random Dance Company's performance that had played to very good houses, identified a number of factors contributing to its success:

> The performance had been in partnership with the region's National Dance Agency [Swindon Dance] performance season 'Taking Risks', which meant that the performance had been partly created at the agency and included in another venue's publicity. But more important was the company's powerful image which the venue had featured on the front of their brochure. The Dance Development Officer contacted a large group of French students who atten-ded....The main reason for success was the product itself, it clicked;

with young people; very accessible, very distinctive and people understood what it was about...the dancers were excellent. Wayne McGregor can de-bunk the myth of a dancer.

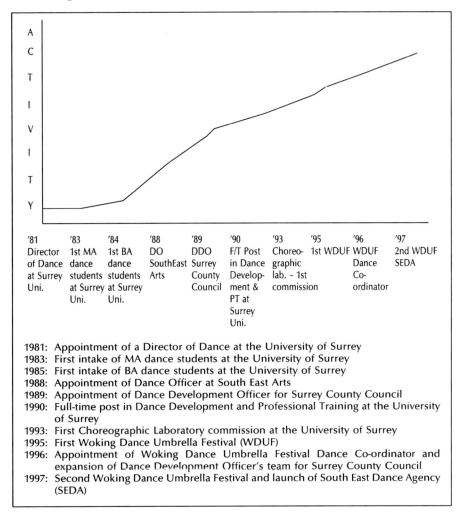

	'81	'83	'84	'88	'89	'90	'93	'95	'96	'97
	Director of Dance at Surrey Uni.	1st MA dance students at Surrey Uni.	1st BA dance students at Surrey Uni.	DO SouthEast Arts	DDO Surrey County Council	F/T Post in Dance Development & PT at Surrey Uni.	Choreo-graphic lab. – 1st commission	1st WDUF	WDUF Dance Co-ordinator	2nd WDUF SEDA

1981: Appointment of a Director of Dance at the University of Surrey
1983: First intake of MA dance students at the University of Surrey
1985: First intake of BA dance students at the University of Surrey
1988: Appointment of Dance Officer at South East Arts
1989: Appointment of Dance Development Officer for Surrey County Council
1990: Full-time post in Dance Development and Professional Training at the University of Surrey
1993: First Choreographic Laboratory commission at the University of Surrey
1995: First Woking Dance Umbrella Festival (WDUF)
1996: Appointment of Woking Dance Umbrella Festival Dance Co-ordinator and expansion of Dance Development Officer's team for Surrey County Council
1997: Second Woking Dance Umbrella Festival and launch of South East Dance Agency (SEDA)

Figure 7.2 Development of a dance infrastructure

Successful dance programming involves a multifaceted approach. In this instance, Random Dance Company's performance was supported by partnerships, effective presentational tools, a good quality product that was relatively well-known and, certainly, the appeal of the artist. Of great importance was the choreographer's direct and 'down to earth' communication with the audience. The venue is working within an established dance infrastructure. In Surrey too there is now a support structure for dance created from a critical mass, built over a period of time, of professionals in post, both within and outside the venues.

Figure 7.2 shows, through the time line, the development of the dance infrastructure that has affected the venues' programmes. In this challenging business, an infrastructure is crucial in providing a context for dance programmes and sustaining confidence and skills in the managers who deliver them.

Various strategies have been identified for addressing the challenges of programming dance. Most are connected with developing the venues' product: the audience. Some audience development strategies are more concerned with broader aims in education, access and raising the profile of the venues as dance centres; others are more obviously marketing led. The weight of these strategies focuses on promoting contemporary dance, as it is the shortage of audiences for this genre that has driven venues and funding bodies to be particularly inventive and creative in their audience development schemes. Not all such strategies lead to an increase in audience numbers. Selling more seats is important, but it is only one aspect of audience development. Participation in dance reaches a different audience from performances, interacting with artists is important for the profile of the venue and securing its role in the dance/arts infrastructure in the country. If there are going to be future products to programme, then some venues will have to provide the space, time and crucial links with potential audiences.

Different people and agencies working together were of great importance to the success of Random Dance Company's performance. Their success on this occasion might offer a way forward for this group of venues.

Networking: a way forward

Financial constraints, concerns over the availability of suitable product, and the drive to improve audience numbers are encouraging venue managers to consider networking as a means of co-ordinating bookings and pooling resources as a marketing initiative. Trevor Mitchell would very much like to see:

> A venue managers' consortium; [the aim is to] get together to bid for
> an amount of money to set up a tour, assist each other with publicity
> mail-outs and help each other.

Partnerships have already been forged through venues working together: for example, Epsom worked with the University on a young artists' commission; South Hill Park Arts Centre and the University have jointly commissioned artists and presented performances; the Woking theatres and the University share mailshots; and the University's programmer is directly involved with the Woking Dance Umbrella Festival. The communication channels flow in and out of the University. Yet there is very little communication directly between the other venues. The University, as a specialist dance centre and the provider of trained professionals and informed audiences, is the engineer of these links; it demonstrates the positive effect that a specialist dance resource can have on an area. The other venues have remained self-contained, to a large extent, only relating to their local funders and audiences.

Yet from the research, a need has been identified to initiate a meeting of the venue managers to take forward the ideas expressed by Trevor Mitchell. Attempts have been made to bring the managers together over specific concerns, such as marketing dance through Arts Marketing Surrey (AMS), which provided marketing assistance for three of the venues through the creation of a dance audience database and a brochure detailing all the dance performances available in the area. This had little impact because of AMS's limited resources and county focus: dance audiences are not bound by county boundaries, and relationships between venues depend on complementary policies and facilities defining relationships, rather than just geographical location. A successful network would require working across a larger geographical area to support organic affiliations between venues and managers, built on dance interest and motivation.

Dance programming in this geographical region is relatively positive because there is a very good balance of venues that are complementary in terms of size, facilities and artistic policies, thus providing a diverse programme of dance for the local population. But of most importance are the individuals employed in key posts, who are excited by programming dance and committed to finding audiences. This support moves dance, which might otherwise be regarded as peripheral, to centre stage.

Appendix 1

INTERVAL PROGRAMMING: Dance is programmed at intervals throughout the year as part of a varied art programme

Strengths	Weaknesses
• ongoing dance presence in venue • audiences able to view dance throughout the year • audiences able to stretch their spending over a year • able to take advantage of availability of a wide range of productions	• resource implications in providing special promotional activities throughout the year • coherence of programme less obvious

DANCE FESTIVALS: Grouping companies together into a specific time period of one to four weeks (e.g. Woking Dance Umbrella festival)

Strengths	Weaknesses
• focus of limited and material resources • high profile for events and venue • high profile for geographical area in which festival is located • audiences and artists begin to expect performances at specific times of year • potential to generate sense of excitement	• resources depleted for remaining programme • lower profile for dance events programmed outside festival • lack of continuity, limited opportunities to consolidate or build audiences • audiences not prepared to attend many events in short time period • choice of artists may be limited due to touring schedules

CROSS-ART FORM FESTIVALS: Dance is programmed into music or general arts festivals (e.g. Bracknell Festival, South Hill Park Arts Centre)

Strengths	Weaknesses
• higher profile for events and venue • attractive to sponsors • potential for audiences to cross art forms	• conflict between dance and other attractions • limited number of dance companies in programme • timing/location may not be good for dance

SITE-SPECIFIC: Artists create work for a particular place, which is usually a non-theatre space (e.g. Rosemary Butcher's *Unbroken View*, commissioned by the Department of Dance Studies's Choreographic Laboratory and South Hill Park Arts Centre in 1995, was performed in The Bracknell Gallery)

Strengths	Weaknesses
• meeting a broader audience through taking dance into different spaces • novelty value in using an unusual space, attracting media coverage creating marketing opportunities • different environment can stimulate audience in different ways • possible new funding partners associated with site • new artistic challenges for creators and managers	• non-theatre site may create safety problems for artists and audiences • problems with venue branding new site • intense operational management making demands on technical and management staff • expense of mounting site-specific work and limited earned income opportunities

SPECIALIST DANCE FESTIVAL: Usually programmed as a feature in an ongoing programme, where programmers use special focus events to achieve a particular aim (e.g. supporting new choreographers through Epsom's 1996 festival)

Strengths	Weaknesses
• raising profile of venue as a committed dance venue • clear audience segments to target • more efficient use of marketing resources	• limited audience to target • heavy programming commitment through intensive research

RESIDENCIES: Different patterns have been used from a whole company in residence for one week to a few months. Normally a residency includes participatory events as well as performances (e.g. RJC residency in Bracknell schools)

Strengths	Weaknesses
• development of relationship between venue and company • prolonged presence in venue allows contact with artists and audience to build a relationship • possibilities for venue to build relationships with education/ leisure participation providers • venue seen as committed to dance	• large investment of human and material resources in managing a residency

References

Arts Council of Great Britain (1993) *A creative future: The way forward for the arts, crafts and media in England*, London: HMSO.

Brennan, L. (1997) *Audience Development an Evaluation and Discussion of the Appropriateness of Horsham Art Centre's Audience Development Policy for Dance*, Unpublished BA paper, University of Surrey.

Brook, P. (1972) *The Empty Space*, London: Penguin.

Marchant, G. (1996) quoted in *Getting in Step: Choreographing the Relationship Between Dance Companies and Venues*. An action plan from the one-day seminar at the ICA, 29 February 1996, Sussex Arts Marketing.

MANAGING DANCE
PARTICIPATION

Introduction

Linda Jasper

Dance is an activity that a large proportion of the population engages in. They do so for a variety of reasons: for health purposes, to socialise, to learn different dance styles, to celebrate an event and for creative or performance opportunities. Dance does not require any other materials or equipment, except for the body: it is a truly accessible activity. The diversity of reasons for participating in dance is reflected in the breadth of contexts in which it occurs: statutory education, leisure and sports centres, hospitals, pubs and clubs, private dance schools and arts centres, to name just a few.

The delivery of dance as a participatory activity is a vibrant and growing industry run by people in full- and part-time funded posts, commercial businesses, and freelance and voluntary workers. The growth of the industry is demonstrated by the expansion in the number of community dance practitioners, who represent one sector of the industry. Community dance is a term used to define subsidised arts practice that is offered within non-statutory education settings for a wide section of the population. It has become a major focus in raising awareness and work opportunities for teachers, choreographers, performers and administrators.

For most individuals their first experience of organised dance participation is in school. Two of the authors in this section, Christopher Thomson and Sara Reed, discuss dance management practice in statutory education, but from different perspectives. Reed presents a case study based on two schools to demonstrate how dance education can be delivered; it illustrates the various factors that influence the development and impact of dance on pupils, staff and the wider community. From the position of an arts organisation, Thomson discusses the management processes involved in 'artists in schools' projects. The dance taught in schools tends to be centred on the 'dance as art' model: the creation, performance and evaluation of dance. It is this model that is exemplified in both Reed's and Thomson's chapters. In contrast, Rebecca Clear's chapter on the leisure/recreation sector emphasises participation and promotes dance as a healthy living model, which encompasses a wide range of activities from theatre dance to aerobics. The adaptability of dance activity in delivering both arts education and healthy living outcomes leads to an ambiguity as to whether it should be placed, funded and managed in the arts or sports sectors. This has been particularly apparent within the education system where it is formally placed in the National Curriculum as part of physical education, but the activity itself may be labelled as performing or creative arts. Dance educationalists have, over many generations, fought for dance to be afforded the status of a separate discipline, which it clearly is. This same ambiguity is causing concerns for the recreational dance and movement organisations of the Central Council for Physical Recreation (CCPR), as described by Clear, which receive funding from the Sports Council. As the Sports Council's work tends to be focused on the élite athlete, future funding for recreational dance and movement is perceived to be uncertain.

In Reed's chapter the use of artists in schools as a resource to augment and enrich the dance curriculum is apparent: pupils and staff can benefit from having direct access to artists to extend their understanding of techniques, choreography and repertoire. Thomson's chapter illustrates how dance artists can work effectively in this environment. Limited opportunities for artists to be employed as dancers and choreographers in the United Kingdom, has prompted them to diversify and apply expertise in other work contexts. As Thomson suggests, many dance artists are multi-skilled, being capable dancers, teachers and/or managers. Many aspects of working as a professional dancer incorporate teaching: the choreographic process, the reconstruction of past works and daily class may all include demonstration, coaching and professional guidance. It is not surprising, therefore, that many dancers work in education and, for a significant number, this is an area of work to which they are committed and skilled. Organisations that train artists to work in education, broker partnerships between artists and educational institutions, and organise projects are extremely important in managing this whole area of dance participation.

Negative attitudes to dance and the dancing body within Western culture have resulted in inadequate financial resources for space, equipment, curriculum time and specialists in the art form. This is in contrast to other areas, such as music and visual arts, which have been embedded within the formal and informal education sectors for many centuries. The National Lottery has provided opportunities, through the capital programmes managed by the Arts and Sports Councils, to build specialist dance spaces. Organisations seeking such funding must demonstrate that the spaces can be accessed by the wider community. In addition, political moves to provide greater parental and pupil choice and raise standards in education have created the Specialist Arts College scheme, which offers funds to enable schools to become 'centres of excellence' for the arts, or other disciplines such as languages, technology or sports. These initiatives have had a direct impact on the two schools presented in Reed's chapter, illustrating a trend that encourages partnerships between education and other sectors in order to provide arts provision for a broad section of the population.

Access to dance participation, regardless of gender, physical ability and economic means, is a policy common to many of the sectors involved in dance participation activities. It is rooted in the belief that it is the right of the individual to be able to partake in dance activity. This conviction is evident in the many determined practitioners whose mission to change perceptions of dance has become the driving force of their work. Dance still depends on people who are prepared to commit themselves over a long period of time to develop work in a particular place, as Chapter 9 illustrates. Yet if an activity is to survive in the long term, it has to become less reliant on charismatic individuals and find an institutional framework. The models for the delivery of dance participation programmes described in this section indicate the various ways in which this might be achieved.

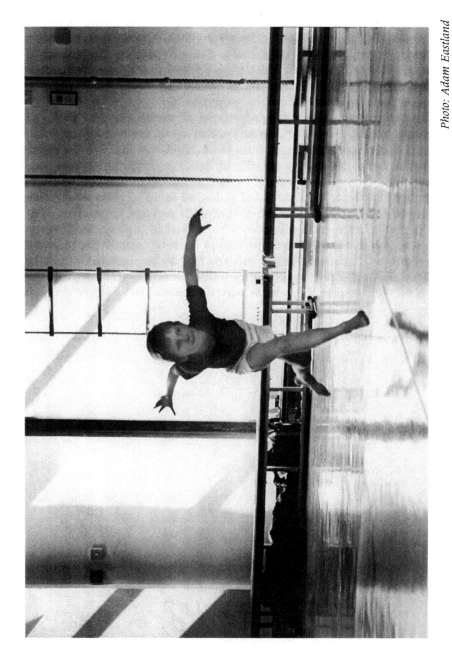

Education & Community Programmes at The Place. Rural primary school residency at Probus School, Cornwall, March '93

8

The Creative Management of Dance Artists in Education Projects

Christopher Thomson

Over the past 30 years a variety of factors and events have led to a professional dance culture in Britain that embraces dance in education and recognises the role that dance artists can play in complementing and contributing to the dance curriculum and extra-curricular education projects. Charismatic individuals, proactive institutions, market-driven reforms, entrepreneurial flair and personal necessity have all played a part in creating a diverse and resourceful dance profession, in which many artists are also highly competent managers. This chapter outlines the history of this infrastructural development and offers some points for reflection on the notion of creative project management.

The recent history of dance artists in education projects began in the 1960s when Peter Brinson, then director of the UK Branch of the Calouste Gulbenkian Foundation, began to promote and to fund 'artists in residence'. The idea was that working artists would set up a professional base at an institution, thus creating a window on their creative life, enriching the host organisation through teaching or collaboration, and perhaps nourishing their own work through contact with the 'real world'. Early 'residencies' saw, for example, a string quartet installed at a university. Soon the idea spread to other art forms and other educational institutions, expanding downwards to secondary and primary schools. The idea also extended to 'community contexts': visual artists, writers and dramatists would use a neighbourhood as their place of work for up to a year, or would make bases at prisons, hospitals and factories, (although this often proved more difficult).

Brinson's original concept had expanded from the idea of a visiting academic. Consequently, several early schemes used the title 'fellow' or 'fellowship', a usage borrowed from the world of the old universities, to describe these resident artists. The intention was undoubtedly educational, but the terminology could be characterised as 'Roman', to borrow Brinson's own description of that patrician attitude to the arts which seeks to pass culture down from a privileged élite to a needy multitude. In time, it would be argued that an 'Athenian' or democratic approach was more desirable and less patronising; but, at the time, the impetus for such schemes was both well-intentioned and timely. It drew on the energy and radical idealism of the 1960s and early-1970s, and linked this to the emergence of a generation of young artists who were not content with the gallery, the theatre or the concert hall, and the audiences who frequented them, but who sought a more direct contact with the world of 'ordinary people'.

Throughout the 1970s, Brinson and the Gulbenkian Foundation assiduously promoted community arts, and funded developments in community dance and dance education. Over the same period, opinion at the Arts Council had grown more favourable to education. Secretary General Roy Shaw had a distinguished background as an educator, and in 1976 a report by Lord Redcliffe-Maud, *Support for the Arts in England and Wales*, argued strongly in favour of the arts in schools. In response to the report, Shaw led a move to decentralise the arts, encouraging artists to base themselves outside London; he sought to develop partnerships through the Regional Arts Associations and local authorities, not only to build their commitment to funding the arts, but also to community development *through* the arts. In 1976, the Gulbenkian Foundation offered funding for the first community dance post, that of Dance Fellow in the county of Cheshire. Veronica Lewis, a choreologist and musician, took up the post and was based in the small industrialised town of Ellesmere Port. She was one of an increasing number of dancers who were looking for ways to bridge the huge gap that existed between dance as taught in schools and dance as art. The intention was to take the best of both and create a new breed of dancer. Since the opening of the London School of Contemporary Dance in 1966, interest in contemporary dance had steadily grown and by the mid-1970s there were more trained dancers than there were jobs with established companies. Small independent dance groups began to form, many graduates became influential teachers, and others sought new ways to combine their dance skills and knowledge with earning a livelihood. Community dance and dance in education began to be elaborated by energetic and idealistic young dancers. At the time they had to administrate their own work and therefore from this period we also see the emergence of the dancer with management skills.

1976 also saw the first 'residencies' by London Contemporary Dance Theatre. The company was based at such institutions as the University of Hull, the University of York, Bretton Hall, I.M. Marsh College and Lady Mabel College, and from these bases dancers and musicians travelled out to work in primary and secondary schools. Following this, and building on a model of dance artists in schools that had been tried out in the USA under the auspices of the National Endowment for the Arts, the Arts Council promoted a series of 'Dance Artists in Education' projects from 1980–83. During this period an Education Department at the Arts Council, initially funded by the Gulbenkian Foundation, was created; shortly afterwards the Dance Department at the Arts Council launched a pilot scheme to establish more dance animateur posts. This was followed in 1983–84 by a national evaluation of the nascent community dance movement; the result was the creation of a national organisation for the development of community dance.[1]

In 1982 the Gulbenkian Foundation had made another timely and important intervention with the publication of *The Arts in Schools*. Though dealing with the arts in general, this study profoundly influenced educational thinking and helped to provide a clear and persuasive rationale for the place of the arts in the school curriculum, as well as giving descriptive accounts of good practice and recommendations for the future.

These developments took place against a background of change in the way dance was taught in schools. Broadly, the creative ('modern educational') dance tradition forged by the followers of Rudolf Laban, and implanted in the school dance curriculum in the 1940s and 1950s, was in decline, at least in some areas. In contrast to free improvisation and individual creativity, a new emphasis was placed on contemporary dance and, to some extent, on dance technique. Although modern educational dance (which had become outdated in much of its imagery and style) continued in primary schools, contemporary dance flourished in secondary schools and higher education. Modern educational dance also lost momentum in teacher training colleges, where the new, young dance groups were performing and offering what had come to be known as 'workshops'. By the mid-1980s community dance and dance in education had become well-established, and the idea of artists in residence had long since broadened from the 'fellowship' idea into a range of project models. These were borrowed in part from the experience and practice of Theatre in Education (TIE), but rather than acting as a medium for learning about social and political issues they tended to place more emphasis on dance knowledge and skills as ends in themselves.[2]

In the late-1980s, the argument for the inclusion of dance in the national curriculum also foregrounded the notion of partnership between dance artists and schools. The idea of 'partners in provision' quickly became common currency, particularly in an already established climate in which most projects were funded from both private and public sources. By the mid-1980s, the earliest community dance projects were so well established that, when the Arts Council's Dance Department commissioned Graham Devlin (1989) to undertake a strategic review of dance policy, several of them became the first National Dance Agencies (NDAs). The aim of these new agencies, as recommended in Devlin's report *Stepping Forward* (1989), was to provide a network of 'safe houses' for dance, offering performance platforms, public classes and workshops, rehearsal space, choreographic initiatives, and support for regionally-based artists.

NDAs have since become a key part of the dance infrastructure in the UK. Simultaneously, a range of other institutional developments has helped lay the foundations for a dance profession that integrates professional, community and educational dance, and one in which dance artists increasingly have skills in teaching and project administration. These developments have included the proliferation of courses and modules in community dance and dance administration at both vocational schools and public sector universities, as well as the introduction of extensive programmes of short courses run by training and management organisations, the NDAs and freelance trainers.

The emergence and growth of development organisations, such as the Foundation for Community Dance and Dance UK, have been another integrating force. These institutions offer information, advice, training and support for dance artists, all of which is predicated on the notion of a multi-skilled dance artist: a dancer with teaching, communication and management skills, who can work in a variety of contexts, and who can devise and manage an education or community project. As a result of these developments a dance profession has emerged with a range of management skills, and a dance culture has come into existence, which broadly accepts that artists can work in education or community contexts without being considered any less skilful, creative or professional than those working wholly in theatre performance and choreography. Artists such as Wayne McGregor (artistic director of Random Dance Company) and Mark Murphy (artistic director of V-Tol), like many others, came to dance through community provision, and see education and youth dance projects as a key aspect of their work. The profession at large is one that has successfully integrated performance and participation, amateur and professional work, project management and the actual business of teaching, choreography and performance. The infrastructure provided by NDAs, development organisations and other agencies, combined with the training and professional development offered by higher education and vocational dance schools, constitute a dance 'ecosystem': information flows well (through listings, databases, on-line services and specialist publications), a range of management training is available, and dance in education and the community is valued by the profession as a whole.

The remainder of this chapter sets out to provide a practical guide to dance in education projects, and to promote the notion that project management can be a creative and learning experience.

Assumptions

We all need assumptions to get by, and to do without them would make project management, and life in general, impossible. As human beings, with a highly developed faculty of memory, we are adept at recognising patterns and making connections. In a given situation we can quickly identify what can be taken for granted and focus on what is new or different. Yet it is a good idea to question our assumptions regularly, especially if we are trying to find out why things are not going as well as they should. Even the most fundamental beliefs are worth examining: does the school actually want this project; do the artists actually like children; and do they even like each other? Sometimes a little amateur psychology is needed: are the teachers feeling intimidated by the artists or vice versa? Such self-questioning can sometimes tell us that 'radical surgery' on a project might be more appropriate than applying a series of 'sticking plasters'. For instance, deferring a residency for a term, in order for it to fit conveniently into the school year, could be better than clinging to the timetable originally planned, even if the change means disrupted arrangements and extra work. Or when a project goes badly, we tend to assume that the funders will penalise us if we admit our mistakes; yet they would usually rather have an honest report so that they, as well as we, can learn from the experience.

This type of questioning is closely related to the idea of 're-framing', which proposes that we should regularly try to see what we are managing from a different perspective. We can re-frame by questioning the unquestioned, by re-examining our strategic objectives, or by adopting the viewpoint of a participant, a member of the teaching team, or a funder. Creative management always involves allowing the possibility that we might have got it wrong, or that there is a better way of doing things: that we can improve the management, and therefore the outcomes, of a project. This style of management treats every project as a learning opportunity for everyone involved. One way in which this can be structured into the process is through our systems of evaluation.

Evaluation

Often, we lurch between carrying out too much evaluation and too little: the former when we circulate dozens of elaborate questionnaires, spend hours analysing and writing up the data, only to send it to the funders and then file it; the latter if we rely on informal verbal feedback (but usually ignore it unless the news is really bad!)

Striking a balance can be difficult, but it can be done creatively and in line with sound management practice. Evaluation starts with deciding what we want to achieve, in line with **SMART** objective setting: our targets should be:

Strategic
Measurable
Apt
Realistic
Time-scaled.

The nature of the event and its objectives should suggest appropriate evaluation methods: these can range from structured observation or conversation, to questionnaires, focus groups or full-scale external evaluation using a number of procedures. Crucially, we need to know what we will do with the results: the value of evaluation is the use we make of it.

At the heart of creative management is the conviction that managing an education project is itself a learning experience. This suggests that evaluation, including monitoring and feedback, should be structured to evaluate the management process as well as the event itself. Importantly though, since the event (or programme of events) should be directed towards strategic aims, the reasons for its success or failure will give us important information about how we manage those aims, in relation to both long- and short-term objectives. Evaluation is a key part of creative management because it embodies our commitment to learning through experience. No manager can afford to stop learning, and evaluation is the structured way in which we reflect on our experience and use that to improve our future practice. Evaluation implies change, and all management is about change in one way or another.

The information that is sought through evaluation serves three purposes:

1. to justify activity to external bodies such as funders;
2. to inform and improve planning and management in the organisation as a whole; and (crucially)
3. to inform and improve the overall programme and similar events in future.

Information can be categorised as broadly documentary (i.e. photographic and video images, text), quantitative (hard facts and numbers) and qualitative (the nature of the experience). Information has to be collected, interpreted, summarised and presented. At each stage we need to know the point of what we are doing, or what we are asking others to do for us.

As with most management tasks, a number of key questions can be asked in relation to the evaluative process: these revolve around the notions of why, what, who, how, when and where.

- **Why** are we evaluating this event? It may be that we have to report on it to the outside world; we want to improve the way we carry out such events; or it will help us to meet our medium- and long-term aims. Preferably all three factors should come into play.

- **What** aspects of the event we are focusing on? Since resources (time, space, finances and people) are finite, we have to be selective in the scope of the study.

- **Who** will carry out the evaluation? In response to this, there are various approaches: systems can be set up that collect information automatically and partners, such as venue marketing departments, can help to collect statistics. One of the most important points for clarification is who has final responsibility for this part of the evaluation.

- **How** will the evaluation be carried out? Perhaps the most commonly used method is the questionnaire. It is important to make forms clear and straightforward, and as short as possible. Effective design can make the questionnaire more readable and user-friendly, and it is worth testing it out on a small pilot group. Standardised questions also allow us to collate information gathered in different evaluations. It is crucial that the questionnaire is perceived as relevant, as the more interested respondents are, the more likely they are to return it.

- **When** should we evaluate? At the end of the session or midway through the season; before and after (to see if we made any difference), and so on. The timing of the evaluation critically determines the type and quality of information we are likely to receive.

- **Where** will the evaluation lead us? In other words, what learning has taken place, and what use will we make of our findings.

All of the above indicate that evaluation is not something to be tacked on to the end of a project or done only because we have to write a final report; instead it should be part of the planning cycle and allowed to change the way we do things, if that is what is needed. Evaluation will inform our own professional development, and our staff training programme if we have one.

Structure and stability

Anyone who has been in a school will recognise that it is an institution that shares characteristics with other schools and has a continuing identity. Schools change of course, but they are concerned to provide a safe, consistent and structured environment in which children (and teachers) feel supported. Routine is part of school life, and managing an 'artist in school' project is, to some extent, about managing the disruption that it will cause to a school. Well-ordered schools can usually cope with temporary changes to their routine, provided these have been planned carefully; they know what to expect and will usually take pride in accommodating the unusual. Over-ordered schools can be difficult to work in and, if they are obsessional about control, this can inhibit children's responses in a creative class. Conversely, children used to externally-imposed discipline tend to lack personal discipline, and therefore dance lessons veer wildly from being over-controlled to being chaotic, so that much time is spent trying to establish appropriate behaviour. Teachers used to tight control can find the free atmosphere of a dance or drama lesson genuinely stressful. Poorly-organised schools may cope with disruption, but life there will be unpredictable, and your project will suffer. An easy-going atmosphere can be appealing superficially, but if it masks a lack of order this will eventually undermine any arts project. The same goes for the management of an artist in school project. Too much structure and there is no room for the unpredictable outcomes that are the essence of art; too little, and there is not enough of a framework to create an ordered and safe space in which creativity can flourish.

Management is often about creating a stable environment in which predictable change (i.e. planned learning objectives) can be brought about: managing instability to create stability. This is necessary for the educational strand of a project. This is not to say that learning comes about only in conditions of stability, but to acknowledge that schools are places where risk usually has to be minimised, and expectations made clear. That said, the artistic aspect of a project can flourish when careful management produces conditions in which outcomes can be unpredictable: managing stability to create instability.

This is partly a play on words of course: each is a facet of the other. Structure is always necessary in an artist in school project. The degree and type of structure, and its visibility or otherwise, vary depending on the scale of the project, the style of the institution, the experience and maturity of the participants, and so on. Structure lets us plan for that uncertainty which we call creativity.

'Vision' and planning for uncertainty

One way to make sure that a creative team is heading in the same direction is to try to articulate a shared vision. In any activity we need a common goal if we are to act in concert, and idealistic aims (a higher vision, if you like) help us to see our immediate activities as meaningful in a long-term way.

Mission statements, the institutional version of vision, are not always so inspiring. By their nature they have to command broad agreement and be 'enabling' statements for the organisation. Yet this can mean that they are so general as to be almost vacuous, especially if encountered out of context. Usually it is the *process* of formulating a mission statement that is most important for the group involved: it is here that common meanings are established and a simple form of words comes to stand for a deeply-felt common purpose. It is not an indelible statement: articulating a vision in this way does not put an end to the need to talk about what we do and why we do it. Visions need to be re-articulated, re-interpreted, renewed. Through this reflection we then re-establish our community with others, the things we have in common and the goals we are all striving for in different ways.

Looking to the future in this way does not mean ignoring the past. Our society is so wedded to innovation (or its shallower cousin novelty) that we can carelessly write off the past as old-fashioned or out of date. Yet our vision of the future is based on what we want to change about the present, and the present is the consequence of what has already happened: we need a sense of history, and a relationship with tradition, in order to envisage the future. Consequently we all look two ways, forwards and backwards, reflecting on our practice and adjusting our vision accordingly.

Sometimes, in managing a project, the 'process' can be allowed to unfold; the vision is not so much a clear picture of what the outcomes are going to be, as a vision of partnership, and of the conditions in which creativity will flourish. The problem with 'process-based' work in education is that if its aims are not clear, the structure and management of the project can be unfocused. One needs to be very clear about being vague! That is to say, certain frameworks and guidelines can allow artists and teachers to let creative work evolve, without needing a clear idea of the final objective. Successful process-based projects are dependent on rigorous and careful planning. Process-based project work suggests that vision can be conceived in a different way: as shared values and a partnership funded on trust. It can allow the vision of a project to evolve gradually because the team has a shared vision:

- a shared commitment to learning;
- clarity about the role of each person in the team;
- trust in each other and in the artistic leadership; and
- a process that involves openness and constant reflection, as structural elements of the project.

It could be described as a 'value-based' vision, in that you do not know quite what your destination will look like until you get there, but as a group you have a navigation system that you can trust implicitly.

This is a sophisticated model and in the context of relatively short-term projects, such as school-based residencies, I would be cautious and say that it is dangerous to assume agreement or mutual understanding. One must be very clear about shared aims and formulate these as painstakingly as any mission statement. It is vital to be clear about roles; have adequate and regular time built in for whole-team reflection and planning; and know that you can trust one another. To achieve this, it is important to be aware of a potential 'culture-clash' between the world of school and professional dance. Time has to be built in to the project planning stage for misconceptions, prejudices and fears that can be identified and addressed. Shared training for artists and teachers can help, preferably with informal workshop episodes in which artists and teachers have to work together on a shared task. Even simple exercises, like describing your working day, what you like and dislike about your work, and the highs and lows of the past week, can help bridge the cultural gap and start to establish the trust on which successful projects are founded.

Key elements of the wider dance/education picture are partnership and trust. These can only flourish where there is agreement (a shared vision) between artists and educators about the kind of world we want to create. Articulating that vision needs time to talk with teachers and, in my experience, that can be hard to find. Teachers are often overwhelmed by the demands of the National Curriculum and its attendant paperwork. Yet it is essential that we have that shared vision, and continue to articulate our reasons for wanting the arts in the school curriculum and in continuing education, at every level. I believe that engagement in the arts nourishes and develops our humanity, that the arts are a large part of what makes life worth living, and that dance in particular should be included in the education experience of young people, both for its intrinsic value and for the ways in which it informs and enriches many other curriculum subjects. A utilitarian view of the curriculum impoverishes and dehumanises young people and their teachers. A school without active involvement in the arts is, in my view, less vibrant, less happy and less self-confident than one which has such involvement.

Such principles may seem obvious, but often they need to be articulated and assented to by team members as part of the management process. Sometimes it is important to highlight them as part of the process of reporting and disseminating project outcomes. For, if the British experience shows anything, it is that project management is facilitated by a culture of understanding: an educational and artistic environment in which the rationale for integration of these two sets of practices and institutions has been articulated, rehearsed and broadly agreed over time. Individual charisma has been channelled by institutional frameworks, and information of all kinds has been stored and made accessible. Creative management in dance education sees each project as making a contribution to these processes and structures, helping to sustain and develop them; unfortunately, they are not self-sustaining in the climate of rapid change that is the defining feature of contemporary life. Project managers, by doing their best to allow for reflection and learning through management structures, articulate the potential, as well as the worth, of dance in education.

Notes

1. The National Association of Dance and Mime Animateurs (NADMA) was constituted in 1986. In 1989 it became the Community Dance and Mime Foundation (CDMF) and in 1995, when responsibility for mime at the Arts Council passed from the dance to the drama department, it was renamed the Foundation for Community Dance.
2. There are some notable exceptions. Ludus Dance Company and Green Candle Dance Company were, and are still, particularly committed to issue-based work and to dance as an agent of social change.

Parts of this chapter first appeared in Thomson, C. (1997/8) 'That Vision Thing', *Animated*, Winter, pp.12–13.

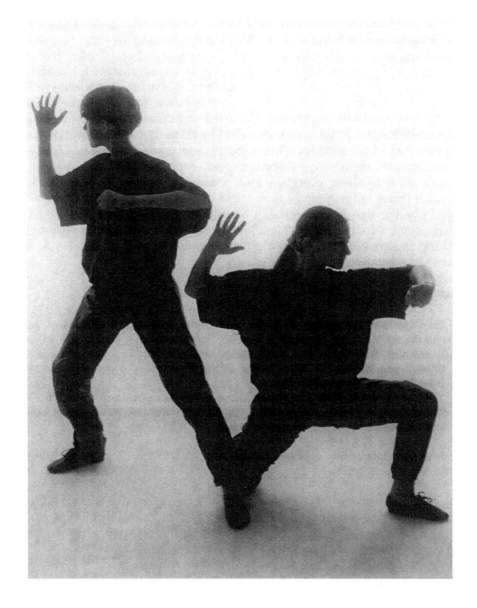

Photo: Glyn Switherman
Dance at Hextable School. Dancers: Carolyn Baker and Christopher Jackson

144

9

Developing Dance in Schools

Sara Reed

This chapter aims to highlight possible models for the development of dance within the formal education context. In doing this, two specific secondary schools have been used as case studies: Stantonbury Campus in Milton Keynes and Hextable School in Kent. These schools have been chosen for several reasons: both have a strong background in dance education; both opened in 1974, and both have applied for Specialist Arts College Status. Specialist Schools are defined by the Department for Education and Employment (DfEE) as being:

> Existing secondary schools which provide rich experiences in their chosen specialism in addition to the National Curriculum. As well as achieving the highest standards in their chosen specialism the government wants them to become a resource for other schools and their local communities.
>
> (DfEE, 1997, p.l).

In many ways these two schools have followed a similar pattern of development; however, due to various factors, the development of dance within each of these different contexts offers an interesting and significant contrast.

The research for this chapter was done between 1997–98 through in-depth interviews with the teachers at both schools, the head teacher at Hextable and dance students at Stantonbury Campus; these were followed up with telephone interviews to clarify information. Documents from the schools and from the DfEE provided another source of valuable information.

Dance in schools – background

Dance education in England and Wales has developed dramatically over the last hundred years; from the late-nineteenth century, when dance was

145

first introduced into physical education training colleges, to 1988, when it became part of the new National Curriculum as a result of the Education Reform Act. Although the statutory obligation is for dance to exist within 'physical education' as part of the National Curriculum, schools may choose to place it within other areas of the school curriculum. For example, dance may come under the umbrella of performing, creative or expressive arts. It is probably true to say that more than any other subject dance has had to fight for its place within the school curriculum. It is recognised, by some well-known philosophers and educationalists such as David Best, Graham McFee, Ken Robinson and Paul Hirst, that dance has a vital and important part to play in young people's education. Yet, in most instances, dance is still the pauper of the arts within the school curriculum.

This raises the question of what dance needs to succeed. Firstly, it requires space; preferably its own warm, clean, and safe environment. Secondly, it must have time to learn physical and technical skills and, like the other arts, time for thought, experimentation and creativity, and time for refining work through practice and rehearsal. Dance often suffers from having fewer hours than any other subject on the school curriculum. In many schools this anomaly occurs because of the positioning of dance within physical education (PE), where time has to be split between the other areas of PE at Key Stage 3 (ages 11–14 years). Dance generally thrives better within a well-established arts curriculum, such as a performing or expressive arts department, where it is recognised as an art form. It is important also that dance is given more curriculum time at Key Stage 3 if students are to develop the skills, knowledge and enthusiasm to be able to progress to studying dance at General Certificate of School Education (GCSE) level (ages 15–16 years) and beyond.

Investment in dance has got to come early on, and support from head teachers, colleagues and governors is vital in terms of providing facilities, finance, space and curriculum time. Dance also needs teachers who are well-qualified and trained and, if possible, visiting artists. The use of dance artists in education is hugely beneficial to the successful implementation of dance in schools, and this is clearly demonstrated through both of the case studies used in this chapter. McFee (1994, p.77) discusses the importance of dance teachers and dance artists in education: 'both have an important role, and might usefully combine in an ideal situation'. These provisions are desirable, if not essential, for the successful development of dance in schools: in the same way that students would not take a science subject seriously if they were not provided with the necessary equipment with which to learn. A lack of basic equipment highlights a hidden agenda, implying that dance is not worthy of proper provision such as that given to physical education or music or science. The cost of providing adequately for dance is often one of the factors that prohibits its development; without the necessary 'tools' of study far fewer students opt for dance than for other subject areas.

In the context of this chapter, it is important to give a brief outline of the funding situation of the schools that are examined. Stantonbury Campus became a grant-maintained[1] school in 1990, in order to retain its comprehensive status when Buckinghamshire reinstated the grammar school system. Hextable School is a maintained school that is owned, funded and operated by Kent County Council through Local Education Authority (LEA) funding. LEA funding comes both from central government and through self-financing. Under the Local Management of Schools (LMS) system, the local authority must give at least 85 per cent of its designated education budget to schools, and this amount is calculated in relation to student numbers. Schools may then decide for themselves how to use this money. The funding for grant-maintained schools is through an annual maintenance grant that is paid by central government through the Funding Agency for Schools; this is calculated so that a grant-maintained school is funded at the same level as LEA funding. Decisions about how the grant is spent and how the school is run are made by the school governors and head teacher, independently of any LEA involvement. The two secondary schools presented as a case study differ vastly in size, geographical location, historical development and funding circumstances.

Stantonbury Campus

Stantonbury Campus is situated within the city of Milton Keynes; it is a mixed ability school of 2800 students, with entry at the age of 12 years leading up to post-16 education for a possible further three years. Stantonbury is unusual in many ways, not least because of its location within the new city of Milton Keynes. The school was created at the same time as the city and its progressive nature and open philosophy owe much to its location and history. Stantonbury is deeply involved in the city's arts and this has been a feature of the school since its very beginnings. The Milton Keynes City Orchestra is situated on campus, which indicates a feeling of partnership between the city, the school and the local community. The school's prospectus states that:

> The arts are central to the achievement of the Campus Purpose, enhancing the education of our students, the work of other schools, and making a vital contribution to the social, cultural and economic development of Milton Keynes.

The school campus includes a professionally equipped theatre, gallery and leisure centre, all of which are used by the community, therefore ensuring strong ties with local groups and businesses.

Stantonbury Specialist Arts College status was conferred in December 1997, with effect from September 1998. The school provides an unusual opportunity for students to be trained and educated to a high standard, not only within specific performance disciplines such as dance, but also in technical and stage management skills, 'front of house' and general theatre management. Up to the age of 16, all of the students study dance as part of a performing arts course, which also includes music and drama. In years eight and nine (ages 12–14) they have three hours per week, with equal time given for each subject; they may also study any of these individual subjects for GCSE. At post-16 level students may study a variety of courses in performing arts, leading to A level qualifications in theatre studies, dance, music and performing arts, or they may join a two-year BTEC (advanced) Performing Arts course.

The campus has two dance studios, one of which is being refurbished as a studio/theatre. In addition, from September 1998, a new, shared, drama/dance studio came into operation. Dance at the school benefits by having well-trained specialist teachers and designated dance studios to work in. The students' dance work is led by a team of two full-time specialist teachers, and another full-time dance specialist joined the faculty in September 1998. This latter appointment has been possible through the funding made available as part of Stantonbury's Specialist Arts College status. Since the targets for this scheme include an increase in the provision of dance at all key stages, an increase in staffing has become essential. For example, the plan states that there should be at least two GCSE and one A level dance groups by September 1998, and three GCSE and two A level groups by September 1999. It also stipulates that all students must follow GCSE course in three arts subjects, and half of those students would take four arts subjects. Vanessa Brown, Head of Performing Arts at Stantonbury, has emphasised how closely the targets must be adhered to in order to sustain funding.

At Stantonbury, as with drama and music, dance students benefit greatly from the programming of performances and events at the campus theatre. For example, there are performance and workshop opportunities given by visiting companies, which in some instances involve other schools and local community groups. It is difficult to separate dance within the curriculum and dance outside the curriculum within this particular context as the two are closely linked; students often work on pieces that are then performed outside school. For instance, the Youth Dance Group and Chance to Dance group are made up of students both at the school and from outside the school, who performed at the Ballroom Blitz festival in London in 1998. This area of work is co-ordinated by Sue Cox, one of the dance specialists who has taught at the school since September 1996. Cox, who came from a career as a professional dancer, was attracted to Stantonbury by the facilities at the campus and by the enthusiasm, respect and support that the arts subjects generate within the school.

Stantonbury is extremely fortunate in having its own professionally equipped theatre, built as part of the school in 1974, which provides a performance venue for student groups, groups within the community, and small-scale visiting theatre, dance, music and opera companies. The theatre is run as a separate unit within the school, attracting funding from Milton Keynes Council, Southern Arts and various trusts and foundations. The school absorbs the cost of salaries for the theatre team, administration, overheads and maintenance. A diversity of work takes place, from the annual dance schools' showcase and regional dance festival, to visits by companies, such as Ludus Dance Company, Mark Baldwin, Ricochet Dance Company, Union Dance Company, Motion House Dance Theatre and Sakoba. Each of these companies have offered workshops, usually involving schools within the Arts Education Forum.

The Arts Education Forum comprises representatives of all the schools in Milton Keynes. Each school belongs to a cluster group and each cluster group has a representative on the forum. Within the forum are music, dance and theatre sub-groups, and it is these sub-groups that deal with the main work; this in turn enhances partnerships with other organisations and schools. An example of the links made between visiting dance companies, the local educational community and the students at Stantonbury can be demonstrated through the residency by Ludus Dance Company, who were at the campus from 26–30 January 1998. This residency was shared with ten other schools, encompassing primary, secondary and special schools, and involved workshops and company and student performances, as well as in-service training for teachers. To make the project financially viable the cost was shared by all the schools involved, and was additionally supported through an award made by the Milton Keynes Community Trust and the Powell Foundation (which promotes access to the arts for people with disabilities). For Stantonbury there were other reasons for its involvement in the residency; the event demonstrated Stantonbury's commitment to sharing resources, thereby helping to meet the criteria set for the school's application for Specialist Arts College status. This relationship with the education sector and the wider community is something that has been developing since the school's beginnings, and is further enhanced through its new status.

Roy Nevitt, the theatre director, has been at the school since its opening, and the development of the theatre, its programming, and the performing arts within the school are all closely linked. This evolution is also inextricably related to the long-term commitment of Nevitt, his team at the theatre, and his teaching colleagues in each of the performing arts areas, with their desire to make their subjects accessible to both performers and audiences. The theatre team comprises the director, two part-time administrators, a full-time technical manager and assistant, and a cleaner. This team deals with all aspects of the running of the theatre. As well as being responsible for the programming at the theatre, Nevitt also teaches A level Theatre Studies and Performing Arts; he sees his role as director of the theatre as being entirely compatible with his teaching responsibilities within the school. This is, very probably, due to the network of support available through the theatre staffing. Sue Cox is involved in the dance programming at the theatre and liaises closely with Nevitt. She is also responsible for liaising with the dance companies who visit the campus, whether at the theatre or the school, or both.

The success of dance, and the performing arts in general, has much to do with a multifaceted system, in addition to a dedicated team of teachers, the facilities at the school, and support from the community, the head teacher, the parents and the governors. The importance of backing from the school hierarchy can not be underestimated. Sally Tyrrell, who has been a dance teacher at the school for the last 12 years, believes that this encouragement is a vital factor in the success and development of dance at Stantonbury: 'the arts are valued, and the injection of money [from its Specialist Arts College status] has given greater kudos to dance.' Tyrell believes that this has a positive and significant effect on the children's attitude to the subject. She has noticed that, with the upgrading of the dance spaces, dance is seen to be important. Tyrell also pointed out that, because students have had to study dance since they arrived at the school, participating in it has never been an issue for them.

It is clear how important it is to the students to have had the opportunity to participate in dance as part of their curriculum studies. They believe that it is important to have dance as a compulsory subject for everyone: 'we wouldn't have known anything about dance if we had not been exposed to it at school.' The students also endorse the value of extra-curricular activities in dance, such as dance performances at the theatre, and highlighted the benefits of being able to perform themselves: 'doing dance and performing it in the theatre has given [us] so much confidence.'

As a purpose-built school, with excellent facilities for the development of dance within a strong performing arts environment, Stantonbury clearly has an advantage. It has built its curriculum around the campus theatre and can therefore provide invaluable opportunities for the enhancement of dance, music and drama within the school. For instance, it can broaden students' knowledge and experience of dance through working with visiting companies, that bring diverse performance and choreographic techniques.

Hextable

In many ways, the work at Hextable is similar to that of Stantonbury School, with the exception that the resources at Hextable are more restricted, due to limited staff provision and lack of suitable dance spaces.

Hextable School is a mixed ability, co-educational, comprehensive school. The school has approximately 800 students and is located in a semi-rural area in Kent. Hextable has one dance studio, with a dance floor and a mirrored wall; the hall can also be used for dance if necessary. Hextable has included dance within its curriculum since the school was founded. At this time it was taught by a PE teacher with a great deal of enthusiasm, but with little experience in dance. Up until 1996 dance came under the umbrella of the PE department, but since then has existed in its own right, as a separate dance department. Pam Howard came to the school in 1979 as a specialist dance teacher, and has been responsible for major developments in dance, both within and outside the curriculum. As the only dance teacher, it has not been an easy job fighting for dance within the curriculum. At Hextable, students at Key Stage 3 receive five lessons of performing arts per fortnight, allocated in the following way: one dance lesson, the same for drama and three lessons for music. Despite this lack of curriculum time for dance at Key Stage 3, the creative and technical standard of dance and the level of dance participation at Hextable is high because of extra-curricular work. Students studying dance at GCSE, A and AS level receive the required curriculum time to follow these syllabi. This is a familiar pattern in many schools that purport to offer dance at Key Stage 3. Another common curriculum pattern in secondary schools, is for students to receive two compulsory blocks of dance over the first three years of secondary school, plus one optional block, each ten weeks. Students may therefore have a maximum of 30 hours of dance over a three-year period.

At Hextable, as at many other schools that offer dance, the dance curriculum is so reliant on extra-curricular dance activities that it could not stand on its own. Howard comments that she feels as if she should not be doing so much in her own time:

> We're not managing to produce the work through the curriculum time well; the curriculum time is minimal and more students would

have a richer experience if there was more time in the curriculum for dance.

Sheila Smith, the Head Teacher, is acutely aware of this problem and increased the time for dance and drama from September 1998 to two lessons every two weeks.

The issue of providing for dance adequately within the school curriculum at Key Stage 3 is an important one; not all children are able to attend extra-curricular activities and in any case, these should be for the *enhancement* of the curriculum, not for its delivery. For many years Howard was the only teacher of dance at Hextable in the post of Head of Physical Education. From the beginning of her appointment, Howard introduced professional dance companies and artists at Hextable as part of the dance curriculum work. She believes strongly that dance could not have flourished so successfully without this input of extra-curricular dance from dance artists and dance clubs which she organised at lunchtimes and after school. When asked about the impact of dance artists' involvement in the development of dance at Hextable, Howard commented: 'to be truthful, I don't think dance would be where it is in the school without that extra involvement.' The cooperation of other colleagues to release curriculum time is crucial to the success of this work.

Howard believes that contact with trained artists and dance at a professional level can give young people an understanding of the creative and technical possibilities of dance. Howard has also used dance artists as a way of providing positive images for boys interested in dance. For example, the students at Hextable have had many opportunities to work with male, as well as female, dancers, with groups such as Phoenix Dance Company and the Jiving Lindy Hoppers; positive male role models are particularly important where female dance teachers are predominant.

The work at Hextable has built up gradually, with greater inter-school collaboration from 1990 onwards. This was due to a project with Rambert Dance Company working with Hextable, Northfleet School for Girls and Kent County Youth Service; the project was supported by funds from Sevenoaks District Council and sponsorship from local businesses. In 1994 Hextable School was integral to the running of a festival for the arts in collaboration with other local schools and colleges. This was organised and run by Focus on the Arts Ltd, a non-profit-making charitable organisation, set up by schools in the area to co-ordinate the artistic activities across North West Kent and to protect, support and encourage the arts for young people in the area. Howard was seconded for one day a week to work on this project, hence Hextable's specific involvement. This and subsequent festivals were vitally important in that they identified the extent of local interest in the arts, and were seen as an important step in the plan to obtain lottery money for a community arts centre at the school. This was an initiative instigated by Howard in 1995 and has been supported by Sheila Smith since this time.

Howard went on to run two further arts festivals at the school in 1996 and 1997, both of which had a strong emphasis on dance. After the 1996 festival Hextable was successful in gaining an award for a feasibility study, for a capital project, from the Arts Council Lottery Fund. In conjunction with this, it was also decided that an application should be made for Specialist Schools status. In making these applications Hextable has had to enhance its activities to develop a community programme that would satisfy the criteria for both:

> Essential to the success of any Lottery funding is a commitment on the part of the school to the community use of its facilities, to be provided for a minimum average of 40 hours per week throughout the year.
>
> (DfEE, 1997, p.20)

> Development plans should include imaginative and coherent plans to share ideas, good practice, facilities, provision, and expertise with other local schools and groups within the local community.
>
> (DfEE, 1988, Annex A, p.l)

The development of a community programme was done through the Hextable arts festivals, a community arts programme of classes and workshops, a greater liaison with local schools, and the formation of the Swanley Schools Consortium, which plays a similar role to the Arts Education Forum described in the section on Stantonbury Campus.

In 1996 Smith appointed Howard as Community Development Officer to coordinate the development of a community programme. Howard relinquished her post as Head of PE but continued as a part time teacher of dance with a newly-appointed part time dance teacher joining her in September 1997. She spent 50 per cent of her time teaching dance as part of the school curriculum and 50 per cent as Community Development Officer. From September 1996 a pilot scheme of community classes was set up and was so successful that a permanent programme of classes, running three evenings a week, was established that offers up to 50 classes including dance, art, music and drama. Since the classes began, the participation has increased; sometimes as many as 500 people attending weekly. A part-time administrator has been provided for the community programme as well as the hourly paid tutors. These are funded through the Community programme. The school also now provides administrative, secretarial and financial assistance for these activities. In June 1998, Howard resumed a full time post at the school as Projects Officer with overall responsibility for dance: 40 per cent of her time will be spent on teaching and 60 per cent on administering a range of projects. A full time dance teacher is to be appointed in September 1998.

Hextable School is now at the centre of two very important and exciting developments: one is their bid to become a Specialist Arts College; the other is the stage 2 of a National Lottery Arts bid. If these developments go ahead then it is certain that there will be much more support in terms of resources. Specialist Arts College status brings with it the initial funds of £200000, which is made up from £100000 raised in sponsorship by the school, and £100000 in matched funding from the DfEE. It also brings additional annual funding based on student numbers, to a maximum of £100000, initially for two years and possibly for three years, depending upon the fulfilment of the annual performance targets set by each school and agreed with the DfEE.

It is significant that these developments have come about through the hard work and extreme dedication of Howard over many years, in addition to the success of the students in dance and the other arts subjects. At Hextable, Howard had to invest much time in gaining the support of the local community, the Head Teacher and her colleagues, before any progress could be made in developing facilities and resources. For years, there had been much outside interest in Howard's work by teacher trainers and dance companies committed to dance education work. Smith does admit that the change to Specialist School status is not without risk, as there is the possibility of alienating some staff, local people and parents. Yet, because of Hextable's strengths in art and dance and the arts in general, her belief in the arts in education, and her experience as an advisory teacher for ten years, she is willing to take this risk. Smith strongly endorses the ability of dance and the arts in general to build confidence in all children, but particularly in those with low self-esteem. As Head Teacher she has endorsed and supported the work of Howard in dance.

For Hextable the granting of Specialist School status would not only provide much-needed new facilities, but would also allow the school to appoint additional specialist teachers and support staff. It was a prudent decision to apply for both a National Lottery grant and Specialist School status in tandem, since at least part of the £100000 sponsorship raised by the school to support its bid, plus the matching DfEE capital grant, might qualify as partnership funding for the schools National Lottery bid.

The two case studies: summary

Both Stantonbury and Hextable have in common the need to expand existing facilities and provision. Yet because of the different context within which Stantonbury has developed, such problems have not been as difficult to resolve. Stantonbury's size, its location in a 'new' city and community which sees itself as forward-looking and experimental, and the attitude of the school itself, have resulted in the school having far better resources than those found at Hextable. It demonstrates the value of adequate support, both human and financial, in providing for dance participation. The granting of Specialist Schools status should ensure that Stantonbury will continue to develop and to broaden its dance participation both within and beyond the school curriculum.

Stantonbury, however, is an unusual context, and a clear example of how resources attract resources. Stantonbury has always had very good facilities, but dance within the school has tended to be taught as an interdisciplinary subject in conjunction with art, music and drama. At Hextable School the development of dance has been restricted through the lack of adequate resources, funding and, until recently, support from senior management. Yet in spite of these difficulties, dance has 'made it', because of the work of Howard. The reputation that Howard has built at the school is recognised nationally within dance education at all levels, by specialist teachers, dance company educators and practising artists. The profile of the school has been enhanced through this, and it is to the school's benefit that dance can lead its bid for National Lottery Arts funding.

Most schools will not be in a position to apply for a National Lottery Arts grant or for Specialist Schools status, however, much can still be learnt from looking at these two models. Schools can benefit from networking with other schools in the area, building links with Specialist Schools and by participating in joint projects where costs and organisational responsibilities can be shared. The schools are not the only beneficiaries of improved facilities and status. The sharing of school facilities within the local community can raise awareness and profile of dance participation in school, which may in turn also attract funding. Working in partnership with local arts organisations may provide projects that include performances by dance companies. School and local business partnerships may result in schools gaining financially, while businesses benefit from publicity and improved profile within the community. Staff, however, need to be aware that it takes time and commitment to develop dance participation and to be able to demonstrate a demand for the subject before support is forthcoming.

These two case studies demonstrate the possibilities for managing and developing dance participation within formal education. Stantonbury may be seen as an extreme and unusual example, and the challenge has undoubtedly been greatest at Hextable. The development of dance at Hextable illustrates what is possible over a period of time within a LEA Partnership comprehensive school. Yet within dance education it should not be necessary to have to fight so hard for what is essentially the right of every child. The examples given here, and the strategies used by the two schools, may help dance educators and school managers to provide the chance for *all* children to dance in their schools.

Sara Reed would like to thank Roy Nevitt, Vanessa Brown, Sally Tyrell and Sue Cox from Stantonbury Campus and Pam Howard and Sheila Smith from Hextable School for their assistance in compiling the data for her case studies.

Notes

1. *Grant-maintained schools*: usually former county, controlled, voluntary aided or special schools that have left Local Education Authority control and become self-governing. They are funded directly by central government through the Funding Agency for Schools.
   Grammar schools: secondary schools open to pupils selected on academic ability; they may be funded by the Local Education Authority, privately or be grant-maintained.
   Comprehensive schools: secondary schools open to all pupils regardless of academic ability, usually funded by the Local Education Authority, but can also be grant-maintained.

Reference

McFee, G. (1994) *The Concept of Dance Education*, London: Routledge.

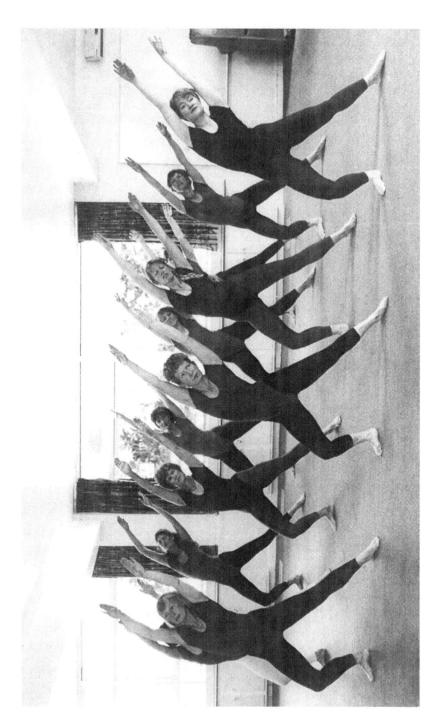

Health and Beauty Exercise

10

Recreational Dance: Issues and Strategies

Rebecca Clear

Dance has always been, and will remain, a social activity. It provides a means of meeting people, making friends, creating and celebrating a sense of community. This chapter looks at some of the challenges of promoting recreational dance, specifically for the sector embraced by the Central Council of Physical Recreation (CCPR).

CCPR is a membership organisation, providing independent representation and a united voice for 280 national governing bodies of sport and physical recreation in the UK. Membership is categorised into six groups of common interest, one of which, the Movement and Dance Division, includes 28 organisations representing recreational dance activities ranging through movement, ballroom, country, fitness, historical and theatrical forms. In the main, the governing organisations provide training for their member teachers, progressive syllabuses, examinations or competitions, special events, information and general promotion. Their teachers offer regular classes or dances in local halls, leisure centres and educational establishments. Some teach on a full-time, possibly itinerant basis, but many teach part-time pursuing very different jobs as their main career. They work as independent practitioners or are contracted by health, community or education agencies. At local level teachers may be relatively isolated; as a member of a national governing body they are part of larger community and have access to the benefits of colleagues, professional development and a sense of belonging.

Funding

While the activities provided by this sector impact on a range of social agendas, notably community development and health promotion, they fall outside the priorities of most public funding agencies. Traditionally CCPR and some of the governing organisations have received funding through the English Sports Council as part of the Council's interest in mass participation in physical activity. Following the poor collection of medals at the Atlanta Olympic Games in 1996, however, the government urged that more emphasis should be placed on the funding of 'élite' sport, i.e. the research and specialist facilities that would enable international competitors to improve their performance. The arrival of the new Labour administration in 1997 brought a partial revival of a 'sport for all' policy, but the emphasis on sporting excellence persists. Such a focus is clearly at variance with the ethos and aspirations of recreational dance, even allowing for the Olympic ambitions of 'Dancesport'. In parallel with this policy development, funding for recreational dance has declined over the last four years. To an extent, the English Sports Council could be seen to be moving closer to the position that the Arts Council of England has always maintained with its focus on artistic excellence. While the Arts Council funded some aspects of participation in dance through its dance animateur and youth dance programmes in the 1980s, these have always emphasised partnerships between local communities and professional dance artists rather than a regular commitment to classes or dances. For the Arts Council, creativity and art takes precedence over social recreation, even though it is recognised that recreational dance has an aesthetic dimension.

Other sources of funding are available at local level. For example, recreational dance teachers could have access to funds from local authorities although, usually, they would have to argue that they are addressing some form of social need. Similarly, individual health, social service, employment, education and prison services may experiment with dance programmes on a project basis. Developing this type of partnership, however, usually involves a significant investment of time, which is rarely available to self-employed, part-time or volunteer teachers. Recreational dance as provided by CCPR member organisations provides fun, social and healthy activity as a part of everyday life; it is more about lifestyle maintenance and enhancement than addressing social need, although it can play such a role in certain circumstances. In common with much preventative medicine, this personal and social maintenance role is often less than attractive to funders.

About 5 million people participate in dance each week (General Household Survey, 1998), and research by the Scottish Sports Council in 1994 found that more people danced than played football, rugby or cricket, or took part in athletics, cycling or running. It could be argued that, as a popular and worthwhile activity, recreational dance deserves funding, particularly at national level where funding could ensure the maintenance of diversity and standards, but there is no-one willing to hear the argument. Evidently then, recreational dance has to rely on its own resources and find ways of being increasingly self-financing. To assist in this, the CCPR's Movement and Dance Division, in partnership with its members, The Colson Trust (a charitable arm of the CCPR), and the English Sports Council, funds the employment of a National Promotions Officer to provide advocacy, promotion and co-ordination for the activities of its member organisations. My own experience in the position of National Promotions Officer informs this chapter.

Issues

A survey of the history of recreational dance highlights many of its current strengths and challenges. Its beginnings were nurtured by a growing concern, at the end of the nineteenth century, with the health and fitness of the population. Movement and dance were considered suitably feminine pursuits and provided an opportunity for women to discover a physical freedom at a time of struggle for female emancipation in social, political and economic spheres. A number of the activities currently embraced by the Movement and Dance Division, which was founded in 1935, can trace their roots to these pioneering times. Significantly, the popularity of formal classes declined during times when women were more fully engaged in national life; for example, during the Second World War which was also a time when social dances were extremely popular, vibrant and physically demanding. Throughout the twentieth century, dance has developed and diversified. In addition to its recreational dimension, it now has a place as a tool for learning in the formal education sector and as a performing art. Increasing diversification and demarcation has brought greater choice and, inevitably, greater competition between the various forms of dance for recognition, status and market share. Fashions in dance forms add a further layer of complexity. The 1990s have witnessed a range of dance crazes including flamenco, salsa, le jive, ceroc and line dancing. The sudden increase in demand cannot always be met and some crazes are short-lived; some expand the total number of people dancing, while others take people away from pre-existing dance activities. Overall, however, a number of the Movement and Dance Division member organisations are experiencing a decline in the level of participation in their particular form.

Image

One of the factors key to a successful operation is the projection of an attractive image. Interviews with member organisations indicate that they suffer from an outdated image. Margaret Peggie of Health and Beauty Exercise (formerly the Women's League of Health and Beauty) sum-marised the problems facing her organisation:

The difficulty lies with our original name and the one we currently use, as well as the perception that we work for older people only: our classes are full of older people who are there because our exercise system is so good [that] they are able to continue into a healthy, fit older age. Our class members were young once and [were] exercising with us. Unfortunately, this is not promotionally attractive. We need an improved name and image, as well as time, time, time and more time, plus financial support of course.

The Keep Fit Association has a publicity committee whose Chairman described a similar image problem:

The media view us as being 'old fashioned' and stuffy. This is proving very difficult to overcome, even with the most dynamic publicity committee I have ever worked with.

As with any lifestyle choice, the image of the activity is a significant factor in attracting new participants. If they perceive a particular activity as being for a different gender or age-group from themselves then they must be particularly brave and enthusiastic about the activity itself, to overcome this image barrier. Consequently the more classes are dominated by older women, the less likely it is that younger people or men will join in. In recognition of this factor, the Keep Fit Association launched a special programme for younger people, 'Youth Moves'. The programme is proving successful, but such initiatives are hampered by increasing demands on the time of young people within and beyond school, including the current emphasis on literacy, numeracy and computer skills, work experience, qualifications and an ever-growing choice of home entertainment.

In a study into the image of recreational dance,[1] 60 Community Dance students aged between 18 and 22 and with backgrounds in theatre dance were asked about their perceptions of recreational dance forms such as keep fit, ballroom and Scottish country dancing. Their response was that, while appreciating the existence of the choice, they would probably not attend such classes or dances which they described variously as unfashionable, unchallenging, embarrassing and reserved for older people. Few had previous experience of the forms they were asked about; where they did have some knowledge it was as part of their studies and therefore remote from the social context. Recreational dance for these students consisted of dancing in nightclubs and at parties.

The most effective route to changing the image of recreational dance is through attracting new participants. This may improve its age and gender balance thereby changing the profile of the participants. Importantly, active participants can be enthusiastic and effective advocates for their chosen dance form.

Potential

Despite its popularity, recreational dance suffers from its isolation, in terms of its position with public funding bodies and its association with a limited participant profile. Both factors can be addressed by re-positioning recreational dance through building links, for example, with the health sector. Dance unites 'doing' with 'thinking' and 'feeling' in a social context. As such it has benefits for the broadest definition of health.

The health benefits of dance are well documented. Disco dancing can increase the heart rate to the same extent as that achieved through a full aerobic 'work-out'. Physical activity produces serotonins, chemicals that create a natural 'high', and it may be assumed that this mood is enhanced by other characteristics of dance such as self-expression and social interaction. Research conducted by the Health Education Authority[2] found that women aged between 16 and 24 were interested in activities that they perceived as 'fun', and involved 'meeting people' and 'looking good', which augers well for the value of recreational dance in promoting healthy lifestyles among this particular group.

The Movement and Dance Division has made inroads into the health agenda, and individual member organisations have participated in health promotion campaigns. This can have benefits for both health and dance, and mutual benefit is the hallmark of all effective partnerships. Some dance activities, however, find their way into the media because they are perceived as injurious to health for example joint injuries, back strain, anorexia; classical ballet being the prime example. While the perception is based on a relatively small number of incidents, and concerns mainly élite performers, 'careful footwork' is required in managing the good news about dance and health.

National promotion

Through the National Promotion Officer's work the membership organisations have benefited from a range of events and services arranged on their behalf. Promotion at a national, generic level is essentially about raising awareness and profile, improving the image and creating a favourable environment for the activities of individual organisations and teachers. These are relatively 'soft' objectives, difficult to evaluate or measure. The inputs, in terms of time, energy and financial resources, are easy to identify but the results are rarely as obvious. Ideally, measures need to be set in advance and to relate to the specific kind of desired change. There are some situations, however, when so many elements are untested or in the control of others that the only option is to 'suck it and see'.

'Dance World' was one such situation. As a national event promoting a wide range of dance practice it seemed obvious that the Movement and Dance Division should be represented. The event, which began in London in 1994, included trade stands, demonstrations and opportunities to participate in 'taster' sessions. Despite being publicised as a national event, the majority of attenders came from the South East of England and, being self-financing through fees paid by exhibitors with profits emanating from attendance charges, the commercial imperative soon became dominant. Over a three-year period the event became a trade show focused on professional dance and lost its relevance and interest for a general public. The particular appeal for the Movement and Dance Division, i.e. the participatory opportunities and the hope that people would continue with activities that they had a chance to try, became less likely.

By contrast 'Ballroom Blitz', an annual festival in London that is part of the South Bank Centre's regular programme, has a clearer focus on participation. There is no entry fee, which makes it highly attractive; people are able to 'encounter' dance with no initial commitment. They can pause and look while they enjoy a drink, and stay or move away as they wish. If their interest is whetted, they can make a decision to attend a performance or talk, or participate in a wide range of dance activities for little or no financial investment. The festival normally runs all day, every day for three weeks and this availability adds to its accessibility. Perhaps most significantly is the association of the venue with 'mainstream' arts activity, which provides a kind of 'kite mark' of respectability and safety. This is coupled with the festive atmosphere, created by the large numbers of people involved as performers and participants, and the inversion of the venue's 'high art' associations as people of all ages, cultural backgrounds and abilities take over the space.

Occasionally the Movement and Dance Division mounts its own events, as it did with 'Spotlight on Dance' to celebrate its 65th anniversary in 1995. This was unashamedly a celebratory event and brought together 500 participants from all over the UK. The audience comprised mainly friends and people already enthusiastic about recreational dance. While it had little impact in directly attracting new participants, it did create a sense of occasion, an opportunity to entertain and build relationships with policy-makers, and to promote 'good news stories' for the media.

The advocacy role of the officer is of great importance in raising awareness of the benefits of movement and dance through placing articles in publications, using media connections and making contributions to conferences. This can identify new partnerships, thereby extending the reach of the CCPR's work.

Local publicity

Generic promotion opportunities also exist at local level and can be more easily followed up, offering greater potential for turning 'intenders' into 'attenders'. A weekend event organised by the Westminster City Council Sports Unit seemed to be designed to achieve just such a situation. A wide range of local teachers were involved, resulting in a broad choice of activities being available. The event was widely publicised and free. It was fun and enjoyable, but failed to attract many people new to recreational dance. It may be that, in this instance, the fact that the event was free led to it being perceived as of little value. Alternatively, it may be that the event was too specialist, with limited opportunities for people to 'encounter' dance other than by making the decision to attend the event. This would be the more worrying scenario for the recreational dance promoter as it would indicate that there is a limited market of 'intenders'; i.e. people thinking they might possibly like to try the activities. The event, however, was successful in attracting primary school teachers who recognised it as a relatively cheap and accessible training opportunity. Secondary benefits can be an effective means of attracting new participants. For example, events held in aid of a charity may attract people more interested in doing something useful for others, and who may, in the process, discover that enjoying themselves is good for them too. A more structured secondary benefit is the Sports Leader Awards run by CCPR which now has a special resource pack to teach leadership through movement and dance. The course provides skills in communication and organisation, together with a recognised qualification and encouragement to become involved in local youth and community activities.

In many ways, at a local level, publicity is the critical process. Local teachers need to publicise their classes and dances in order to inform and attract participants. The best way to convince people that recreational dance can enhance their lives is to get them dancing. The usual means of getting them there in the first place are posters in local libraries, leisure centres and shops. Such publicity need not be glamorous to be effective, as long as it is clear and includes all the necessary information. Home-made publicity material, however, does little to improve the image of recreational dance in general, and it may be that there is a national role in providing local teachers with the tools and material to enhance their publicity efforts.

The future

Securing the future for the present diversity of recreational dance will require continuing promotional activity. Better co-ordination between local and national promotional activity is more likely to succeed than a fragmented approach. The organisations understand the need to improve the image of recreational dance; yet few have reached the stage of changing attitudes at executive level which would produce the strategies and devote the resources essential to bringing about change. Organisations need to identify and segment their market and to target their publicity and promotion efforts accordingly. This means redirecting resources rather than finding new ones, but lack of resources is frequently cited as hindering change. In identifying new markets, young people are often seen as key, as they are perceived to offer long-term potential. Yet the population is growing older and the need for activities for older people may increase as a result.

Recreational dance, as encompassed by CCPR's Movement and Dance Division, has proved itself to be enduring for almost 65 years. This success suggests that the organisations have been effective and flexible in promoting themselves and responding to a changing market. The challenges that now face these organisations are more complex and require a systematic approach. A slow, progressive reorientation from the core of the organisation is needed to reposition recreational dance as an accessible, relevant and health-promoting activity for the new Millennium.

Notes

1. The Liverpool Project promoted by the CCPR Promotions Officer with dance degree students at Liverpool John University in 1997.
2. 'Active for Life', a research project focusing on young women, conducted by the Health Education Authority. Final stage 1998/9.

MANAGING DANCE POLICIES

Introduction

Jeanette Siddall

Previous chapters have dealt with the management processes involved in dance creation, presentation and participation. This section looks at how policies emerge, how they influence the operating environment, and how they can be managed for the benefit of dance. It takes English regional and pan-European examples of policies and explores their impact on the dance landscape.

The landscape is necessarily political, in so far as it is inhabited by cultural practices substantially reliant on government investment. In England the main source of such investment is through the arts funding system. This routes 'grant in aid' raised through the taxation system and funds generated from the National Lottery through the government Department for Culture, Media and Sport to the Arts Council of England, and from there to artists, arts organisations and the ten English Regional Arts Boards. In the other countries of the United Kingdom, cultural funds are routed through the relevant government office. The Regional Arts Boards are autonomous bodies and, while the majority of their funds comes from the Arts Council, they also receive funds from the local authorities within their region and other funders such as the Crafts Council, British Film Institute and others. In addition to funding through this system, artists and arts organisations may be funded by their local authority, urban regeneration schemes, and other public authorities such as for health or education. If they engage in activities outside Britain, they may become eligible for funds from the British Council, which is financed through the Foreign Office, and partnerships with organisations based in other European countries may elicit European Community funds.

The picture is complex and, given that public funds are inevitably subject to public scrutiny measures designed to serve a wider political agenda, the picture is always in flux. Art and politics co-exist in a dynamic, ever-shifting world. Recent examples of such shifts can be seen in use of Lottery funds. Britain's National Lottery began in November 1994 with the arts nominated as one of five good causes to benefit from its proceeds. At that time the major concern was with 'additionality', a criterion that was intended to protect the grant in aid from being replaced by Lottery funds, by clearly delineating these funds as being for 'additional' activity. Initially this was relatively simple; grant in aid was for revenue funding while Lottery was for capital purposes. Within two years the government issued new financial and policy directions to enable Lottery funds to be used for revenue purposes, therefore 'additionality' could now only be maintained through clearly identified schemes. Grant in aid suffered annual cash standstill and small reductions which, with the cumulative effect of inflation, resulted in a significant decline in real terms, and a concern with 'additionality' was replaced by the urge to 'integrate' the two funding streams. A new Lottery Bill was enacted in 1998 that facilitated this change and established a sixth good cause to benefit health and education.

The Lottery brought a new reality to the notion of the people's money. It could be argued that taxation is as much the people's money as Lottery profits, and further that the people have no choice about paying taxes whereas there is no compunction to buy Lottery tickets. Yet the consciousness and tangible nature of the act of buying these tickets creates a sense of ownership about the destination of the proceeds, which is less frequent in the context of taxation. From the beginning, the media fed this interest with controversy, and centred on any Lottery awards that could be seen to benefit less deserving minorities, be they individuals from whom 'heritage' items were purchased, minority social groups, or national opera houses.

Public interest in arts funding in England further increased with the arrival of the new Labour government in May 1997. One of its first acts was to change the name of the responsible government department from National Heritage to Culture, Media and Sport. This signalled a new government agenda and a commitment to engage with the cultural industries in new ways. Radical reviews were initiated, focused on the bastions of the arts establishment. Precisely how radical, and indeed how long-lived, the results of these reviews will be may only be determined through the lens of history. In the meantime, it can be predicted that these will not be the last changes in the direction, ethos, priorities and structures of arts funding.

In a world as influenced as any other by the need to think globally and act locally, this section begins appropriately with the regional perspective. Nikki Crane explores some of the policy issues pertinent to dance development from the position of a Regional Arts Board. She highlights the resources available to such a body, in terms of funds, influence, partnerships, networks and the key role played by individuals working on the ground. With a focus on the experience of working closely with

Suffolk Dance, the National Dance Agency based in Ipswich, she describes the growth in interest, activity and confidence in dance over recent years.

Sophie Lycouris looks at a policy that was not designed to promote dance, but which has great potential for dance. She examines the post-Maastricht European funding context, including the availability of funds for purposes other than solely cultural benefit. She argues the need for dance managers to respond positively and creatively to such opportunities. While the European Union has no policy that deals specifically with dance, it has needed to place an increased emphasis on cultural issues as it has progressed from its early days as a purely economic union. The free circulation of cultural products in itself changes the nature of the cultural identity of individual member states and the nature of the Union. Growing realisation of such dynamics has given culture a new significance in the European integration project. The debate about whether a 'European culture' is discernible or desirable continues, and the Maastricht Treaty recognises the need to promote the cultures of member states while supporting manifestations of a common culture and cultural co-operation. Significantly, the Treaty identifies the need to take cultural factors into consideration in all areas of policymaking. Sophie Lycouris describes approaches and strategies to assist dance managers to make the most of these opportunities.

Dance management is an international business. British dance has a European market and, as Julia Carruthers noted in an earlier chapter, for some artists it is friendlier than the home market. Sue Hoyle contrasts her experience of dance in Britain and France, and considers how different dance policies have both shaped and responded to different environments in the approach of funders, promoters and audiences. She positions dance as a significant promoter of 'people to people diplomacy', with the capacity to make a real difference to the way in which Britain is perceived overseas.

Sue Hoyle concludes this overview of issues and strategies for dance management on an optimistic note, highlighting the potential for dance in a new world. It is a fast-moving world in which cultural concerns underpin political aspirations, are at the forefront of social and economic agendas, and signify and promote our understanding of ourselves and of others. The opportunities are here and all around. The challenge for dance managers is to navigate their way through the opportunities, to develop the confidence to influence policy-makers and to make the support structures work for them. As Sue Hoyle states, 'dance is about people, not products', and it is people that make things happen.

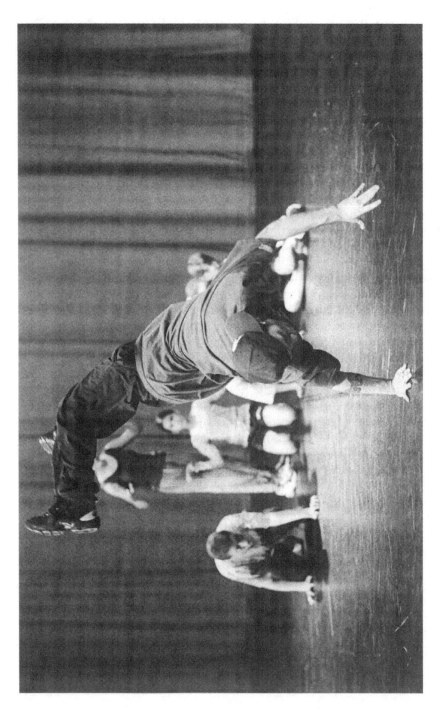

Photo: Mike Kwasniak

'Banksy' working with young people during Suffolk Dance youth summer school, 1998

11

Making Connections: Dance Development in the Eastern Region

Nikki Crane

Introduction

During the early 1970s, dance within the community was centred around a few pioneering individuals who came to be known as 'animateurs', and whose activities were designed according to their knowledge of, and relationship with, the local community. In 1976 there were just three dance animateurs, but this number has now grown to some 600 across the country. From these beginnings, dance in the community has become one of the success stories of the last 20 years and is an area in which Britain is a forerunner.

By the mid-1980s, much had been achieved in creating access to dance; animateurs throughout the country had made vital partnerships with schools and communities, and had made links with sectors as diverse as social services, health authorities and sports organisations. The animateur movement had proved critical in bringing together community and professional practice and in influencing dance education, training and performance. Thus, dance began to make an important contribution to the social welfare of communities. Although some animateur posts had begun to expand into larger community dance organisations, many of these were still operating in isolation, without coherent networks.

In June 1988, I moved from my post as dance animateur for South Humberside, based in Scunthorpe, to become Dance Officer for Eastern Arts Board (EAB) in Cambridge. I was as passionate then, as I am now, about the value of animateurs, and during my interview at EAB I argued that a major step in dance development would be the creation of a regional network of animateurs. As it turned out, it was a meeting of minds. EAB had already established a handful of animateur posts in the region, had seen the remarkable return on its investment in terms of education and continuous development at grass roots level, and was keen to develop this strategy further. This chapter traces the development of dance networks in the eastern region of England; a process with which I have been closely involved over the last ten years. It is important to note that these developments have arisen within a national context, which accordingly forms part of the focus.

As Regional Arts Board (RAB) officer for a seven-county region, with a population of six million distributed between widely dispersed rural areas and dense urban centres, the first problem was how to create a suitably responsive network of animateurs. For example, how could I create a receptive environment for dance in rural Norfolk, complete with its farming communities and fishing villages, compared with urban areas such as Luton, near London? Not only would these areas require different artistic treatments, but there was also the problem of funding. Just as communities often have very differing views as to the importance, relevance and content of art forms, so do their politicians, who regulate major sources of income. Animateur posts, and similar community-based dance organisations, are funded by a complex array of contributions from city, borough, district and county authorities, RABs and private sponsors. Thus the growth of the animateur movement was dependent on the success of the partnerships between these bodies.

First steps in regional dance development

During my first three years at EAB, an immediate priority was to increase the number of animateur posts to at least one per county, in order to achieve an even geographical spread. This was quickly accomplished with the enthusiastic support of local authorities, many of whom recognised the social impact and economic viability of animateur work. It is extremely attractive to local authorities that the cost of importing a professional company for a week's residency is comparable to that of contributing to a local dance agency for an entire year.[1]

The next step in the strategy was to secure further funds from EAB and the relevant local authorities so that some animateurs could expand their operations from local to county level. These larger organisations, known as agencies, were also evolving in other areas of the country, bringing about a shift of emphasis in the role of the animateur, from that of dance-practitioner to dance-manager. There was now the opportunity to promote a high level of networking between EAB, its agencies and its animateurs; this created a 'critical mass' that could replace the somewhat fragmented and low-profile operations hitherto. The network soon began to demonstrate the potential for sharing resources and expertise, minimising duplication and providing the outside world with a clear sense of regional cohesion. In addition to regular contact, we set up a forum that met four times a year to plan and implement training and set out regional dance policy and strategy.

The maintenance of a stable network of dance agencies and animateur posts throughout the eastern region relied on the continuous financial support of some 30 local authorities, whose outlook necessarily tended to be area-specific. Within an often fluctuating political environment, this was a time-consuming business, but one that paid off; local authorities recognised both the value of their own animateurs and began to see the added value of the network.

In 1988, there were no well-established professional companies or resident artists within the eastern region, as is still the case. While it is a longer term aim to rectify this situation, it has provided another incentive to create an infrastructure of dance agencies and animateurs regionwide, consequently, there are now opportunities to establish partnerships, both short- and long-term, with a range of visiting artists. The region benefits enormously from this flexibility and is in a position continuously to assess artists' potential and their relationships to audiences. Simultaneously, artists can benefit from a supportive environment both in terms of local provision and opportunities arising from the network.

The evolution of a strategy for dance

The eastern region dance strategy has been developed in partnership with all the representatives of the regional dance constituency. During the consultation process, it was agreed that our chosen objectives would remain flexible enough to respond quickly in a rapidly changing environment. It was decided that three principles would drive the emerging regional dance strategy.

1. To establish a vertical continuum between grass roots work in the community and professional artists. In this way, we set out to foster standards of excellence at local level, stay in tune with national dance developments and provide artists with a receptive environment for their work.

2. To develop a horizontal continuum of partnerships between the agencies and their neighbouring promoters in order to stimulate and co-ordinate dance programming. It was also important that these partnerships expanded to embrace other regional agencies and organisations involved in dance development. The region's involvement with Eastern Touring

Agency is a case in point. Here, this pioneering agency has been a key player in commissioning and touring dance, supported by tailor-made education and marketing initiatives, to over twenty small-scale venues within the region.

3. To create a climate of autonomy so that the agencies and animateurs, together with other EAB-funded dance organisations, could determine their own artistic direction. The debate about how much influence the various funding bodies should have over clients' artistic decisions, is one that continues to rage. As far as the dance strategy was concerned, however, my contribution was to design efficient structures, and act as adviser and advocate, thereby encouraging organisations to be self-sufficient.

To date, the regional dance agency network, now the largest and most established in the country, comprises five county-wide agencies with 15 personnel and five animateur posts. At the hub of this network now stands Suffolk National Dance Agency (NDA), one of eight such national dance agencies within the country. The following section looks at how this national infrastructure of agencies came about and how Suffolk NDA and the eastern region have developed a unique partnership.

Taking strides: the emergence of the National Dance Agencies

In the late 1980s, the need to develop a more formal national dance infrastructure had been agreed as a top priority by the dance profession and the Arts Council of England. Following Graham Devlin's report *Stepping Forward* (1989),[2] the Arts Council took the initiative to establish a number of NDAs, geographically spread across the country, as part of a ten-year plan. In the report, Devlin articulated the view of the dance profession that NDAs could take a number of forms. Building on the successful work of animateurs, the remit would cover education, information, advice, strategic initiatives and the dissemination of best practice in specific areas of dance. With the large investment of central Arts Council funding, the significant difference would be a greater shift towards the development of the artist and high calibre professional programming within local communities, thus enhancing grass roots activity.

Individual organisations, with the support of RABs, were invited by the Arts Council to apply for funding towards their establishment as a NDA. EAB proposed one its most successful dance agencies, Suffolk Dance, for NDA status and was awarded this in 1993. The application paid particular attention to the potential role of Suffolk Dance in regional, as well as local and national, development. With effective networking under way, the region was in need of a focus for establishing high profile and far-reaching partnerships.

Suffolk National Dance Agency

Suffolk NDA, based in Ipswich, began life as an animateur post in 1983, occupied by Scilla Dyke and, under her leadership, developed by 1988 into a county-wide agency. Thus Suffolk NDA evolved in a stepwise fashion and now, under the directorship of Jane Mooney, remains a model of best practice. There are just four full-time and one part-time staff to manage a comprehensive and demanding programme that includes the production of new work, collaborative international projects, professional training and development, community provision, local authority liaison, and advocacy. It also provides resources and advice locally, regionally and nationally. In addition to the five members of staff at the Ipswich base, there is an animateur post based in Haverhill, specifically serving the St Edmundsbury area.

While animateurs were funded primarily by local authorities and RABs, bringing with them differing principles and requirements, the NDAs were destined to have an additional portfolio of funders including the Arts Council of England, private sponsors, trusts, foundations and, in some cases, European and lottery funding. Such a complex mix of revenue and project funding has placed the NDAs under considerable pressure. The different emphases placed by funders on access and innovation represent just one of the dilemmas. For example, the Arts Council's primary interests are in innovation and dance as a professional art, while local authorities are fundamentally concerned with access and the social impact of the arts. The RABs, funded both by local authorities and the Arts Council, are caught somewhere in the middle. Similarly, with one-off projects funded by different trusts, foundations and sponsors, there are also specific criteria to satisfy. It is in this arena that conflicts can arise, but if handled sensitively by RABs and others, the resulting settlement produces a balanced approach to dance, which is led by both artist and audience, thus satisfying the requirements of all funders. Suffolk NDA is not immune to these difficulties and Figure 11.1 provides a snapshot of the complexities of its financial base.

Navigating through all of this requires agility and any dance agency needs a strong board of management to steer its course. It is in this forum that representatives of the funding bodies can be heard, a consensus can be found and decisions made in a way that keeps all partners on track.

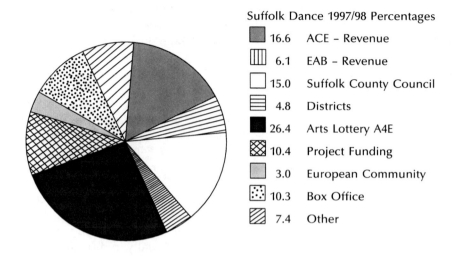

Suffolk Dance 1997/98 Percentages

▨	16.6	ACE – Revenue
▥	6.1	EAB – Revenue
☐	15.0	Suffolk County Council
☰	4.8	Districts
■	26.4	Arts Lottery A4E
▧	10.4	Project Funding
▨	3.0	European Community
⋮	10.3	Box Office
▨	7.4	Other

Figure 11.1 Pie chart illustrating major funding segments (%)
for Suffolk NDA during 1997/98.
Note: In this financial year Suffolk NDA made 44 applications, half of which were successful.

A typical board will include members who can give specialist advice in areas such as artistic programming, fund-raising, financial management, marketing and legal matters. Similarly, dance professionals recruited to agencies now need business acumen, management and communication skills. Unfortunately, too few are equipped to tackle these demands, which raises the question of how best to provide appropriate training in such a fluctuating funding environment.

Current trends in funding

Due to the change of government in 1997, major alterations to the arts funding system in this country are imminent. There is much speculation on how the Arts Council, RABs and local authorities will be affected, but there are indications of a radical shift of funding and responsibility from the centre, via the regions, to the most local levels. What is eminently clear, is that the trend towards multiple funding for the arts will continue as no-one wants to be in the position of sole finder.

As far as local authorities are concerned, there is an increasing trend towards project funding, which allows them greater control, and this would appear to align with the Government's view. High-profile project funding from the National Arts Lottery has reinforced this trend; since its inception, money from the lottery has only been available for capital costs and short-term projects, rather than for core operations. Any competitive funding system creates the possibility that its recipients become vulnerable to the whims of their funders. The danger for less experienced dance agencies is that, eager to secure extra subsidy, they attempt to assuage potential funders, resulting in the disintegration of the organisation's 'raison d'être'.

Long-term planning for organisations is continually hampered by cuts in budgets and the inability or unwillingness of funders to commit beyond an annual agreement. In Suffolk NDA's case, county and district funding currently exist on an annual basis and, while three-year agreements are in place with the Arts Council and EAB, the organisation is still left uncertain as to the exact level of annual funding. An encouraging development is that some local authorities within the region are now looking at the possibility of offering three-year commitments to their clients.

Over the last 20 years, government has expected the arts to become more financially independent of the public sector and, with the new Labour government, this policy looks set to continue. Concerns have been expressed by many leading figures in the arts world that we lack the degree of private sector funding that occurs in many other countries. There is, however, a great deal of untapped potential in developing more imaginative partnerships with business, which is less about cash sponsorship and more about exchanging skills and resources. In summary, the dance agencies must, to some extent, run a commercial operation in order to survive, inject enough innovative activity to satisfy their artistic remit and simultaneously contribute to the social well-being of the community.

Nationally, it is clear that while county council funding for the arts is diminishing, district funding is on the increase. Fortunately, the district councils are generally much larger contributors to the arts, therefore the net effect is that the total amount of funding is increasing. Suffolk NDA is at the forefront of developing effective partnerships with the 'up and coming' district authorities. In order to keep a tight rein on its own aims and objectives while satisfying the requirements of the three district authorities that support it, Suffolk NDA has established 'district dance development plans'. These are contractual arrangements, reviewed annually, designed to explore new ideas and to bring clarity to their negotiations.

As with the animateurs, the benefits of 'buying in' to an agency such as Suffolk NDA, soon become evident to district authorities as they realise that for a small investment (typically between £1000–7000), not only are they gaining work specifically delivered in their own priority areas, but they can also enjoy the 'spin-offs' of being part of a county, regional, national and international organisation. Suffolk NDA has now moved into a position in which it has real bargaining power, as the local authorities look for direction and a sense of cohesion in developing dance. The dance development plans of Suffolk NDA represent a major breakthrough in trying to create continuity against the background of short-term funding.

Presently, the indications from the Labour government are that every local authority will have to produce a local development plan specifying their artistic intentions. No statutory obligation to deliver these specific objectives will be imposed, but the local authorities will have to declare, and more formally account for, their plans. If this materialises, then hopefully there will be greater clarity in the system and better planning, which will assist the dance agencies in developing strategies. These new proposals may well introduce a healthy element of competition among the local authorities.

Communication and advocacy

It has always been a priority for the regional agencies and animateurs to establish strong working relationships with their local authority arts development officers. The number of these posts is now increasing and contributing significantly to the infrastructure at a local level. Thus, if we are to avoid duplication and amass our resources, communication between all parties will need to be even more effective. A model partnership is currently under way in Lincolnshire where the county arts development officer, David Lambert, has worked closely with EAB, Suffolk NDA and the local dance community in devising a dance strategy for the county, which specifically targets district funding. Against the current trend, Lambert has been instrumental in obtaining a 100 per cent increase in county council funding for dance over the next three years.

In the past, the need for advocacy in dance has often been seriously underestimated by the profession, not least animateurs and agencies. It was as though a commitment to the social impact of dance was incompatible with undertaking a public relations role. Times have changed; the precarious patchwork of funding is held together as much by effective business and communication skills as by artistic endeavour. In spite of this, there is still a tendency within the arts towards the correctitudes of overly precious and jargon-laden language that can be alienating. There is no better remedy for this than working with sponsors and the media, as both demand succinctness and a more worldly approach.

Bringing artists and audiences together in the eastern region

In the eastern region we work hard to ensure that the development of artists happens in tandem with the development of audiences. The region has invested a great deal in setting up the existing networks and partnerships, bringing together dance agencies, venues, marketing and education specialists, and funding bodies. It is our view that artists are part of this enterprise and can benefit enormously from such a receptive environment.

The strength of the existing regional networks testify to the commitment to work in partnership. Therefore we can only hope that the artists, with whom we choose to work, will also bring a spirit of partnership to the region and take full advantage of the resources and expertise within the infrastructure. On the whole, this is the case; however, there are still instances in which artists are only too quick to take advantage of the tour bookings on offer, but become reluctant partners when the negotiation asks something of them. There are cases where productive partnerships are set up by company administrators, who generally have most contact with the region, only to be overturned by the artistic director. Consequently, artistic decisions are taken which, to the detriment of dance development, ignore the contributions of regional infrastructure.

Two other major factors threaten the progress of the artist and development of the audience:

- an obsession with innovation; and
- the funders' over-reliance on the crude statistics of quantity.

Innovation is a relative business. What is 'cutting edge' for rural Norfolk may be positively 'safe' and outmoded in London. In the rural areas of the eastern region, touring dance, whether it is 'cutting edge' or mainstream, is a risky business. There are no short-cuts to building audiences. It is a slow process of education and of building trust, so that audiences are not pushed towards the more abstract or esoteric forms of dance too soon. One of the strategies we have adopted is to identify 'safe houses': key venues which have a more developed audience to draw upon for the presentation of experimental work. We ensure that work of this nature is strongly supported by initiatives, such as workshops, talks and debates, designed to maximise interaction with audiences. Building audiences in rural areas is particularly costly and time-consuming, and the problem is compounded by inadequate public transport. Word of mouth and befriending the parish council will, in many cases, be much more effective than a glossy publicity campaign.

Over the years, research into audiences in the region has provided us with vital information for the development of dance, resulting in some radical changes in our approach. We have had to respond quickly and be prepared to change tack as the 'habits' of audiences change. *Map East,*[3] a market research project for the east of England, suggests that contemporary dance attenders would often come to one performance and, thereafter, not return. Consequently, venues have had to meet the challenge of reactivating lapsed attenders.

The same research provided another revelation about regional dance development:

> Funders, local authorities and venues alike had believed that audiences in the east of England habitually travelled for well over an hour in order to attend arts events. This had led to an ingrained belief that the region's venues competed with each other for a large proportion of their audiences. *Map East* demonstrated unequivocally that almost all current attenders came from within a 45-minute drive time of the venue.

The explosion of this myth was to have a dramatic effect on venues' marketing campaigns, as they could now concentrate their limited resources on the real, rather than imagined, catchment area.

Partnerships between dance agencies and venues are crucial to dance development. In Suffolk, many of the venue managers, marketing and education staff look to Suffolk NDA for additional advice and support in devising programmes and creating audiences. Suffolk NDA has responded by establishing the Suffolk Dance House Network; a centre for communication with venues of all scales. This forum assists in the effective co-ordination of dance activity across the county and acts as a catalyst for shared programming, marketing initiatives and education work.

The impact of Suffolk National Dance Agency

Suffolk NDA has created a focus for the regional dance network and has been pivotal in creating imaginative partnerships regionwide. It is now initiating management practices that can be emulated in other areas of the arts and commerce. The achievements of Suffolk NDA are all the more remarkable given the largely dislocated rural environment in which it coordinates its activity. Seizing the opportunities that arise from this, the organisation has pioneered new ways of working in rural areas, for example, by exploring unconventional performance spaces such as Orford Castle, sheltered housing and village halls. Chiefly due to the impact of

Suffolk NDA and other regional agencies, there is now a significant increase in the number of their students returning as professionals and, for the first time, artists from outside the region are seeing the benefits of taking up residencies here.

While Suffolk NDA is recognised by EAB as a centre of excellence in the region, it is essential to realise that the whole enterprise depends on the contributions of all the components of the network. The intention has been to create a climate of interdependence regionwide. As Suffolk NDA increasingly becomes a mentor for regional dance development, both Jane Mooney and myself are committed to ensuring that our roles remain complementary.

The future

Investing in a regional infrastructure in which opportunities for partnerships can flourish has paid off. It is vital, however, that we continue to work on creating synergy between the infrastructure and its artists; each must understand the scope of the other's functioning and resources. Thus the eastern region will inaugurate further training and development programmes to nurture artists within the infrastructure so that they can derive the maximum benefit of its resources. The aim is to think beyond dates and performances and to look at development in a more creative, long-term way. In particular, we will encourage artists to develop track records in their specialities and devise even more effective ways of ensuring that promoters, marketers, educationalists, agencies and artists exchange ideas and learn from each other.

Nikki Crane wishes to thank Adrian Pini, Fred Brookes, Jane Mooney, Scilla Dyke and Lynne Williams for their advice.

Notes

1. A week's residency with a typical small-scale dance company can cost between £3–6000.
2. Devlin, G. (1989) '*Stepping Forward: some suggestions for the development of dance in England during the 1990s*', Arts Council of Great Britain.
3. The research for *Map East* was undertaken by Heather Maitland of Eastern Touring Agency in 1993. It is one of the largest ever analyses of arts attenders.

The views expressed in this article are not necessarily those of Eastern Arts Board.

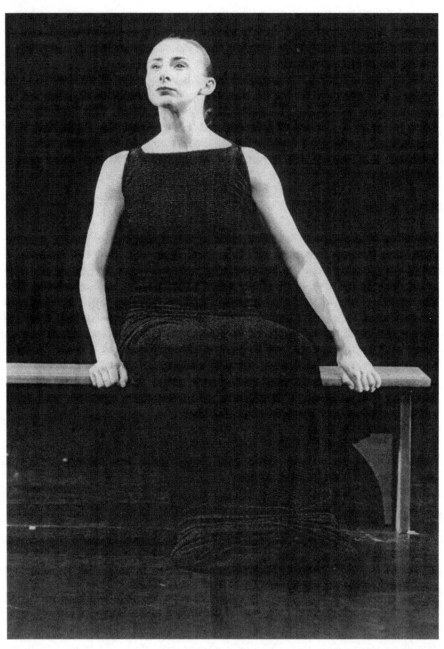

Annamirl Van de Pluijm

12

Post-Maastricht Europe: Challenges and Strategies

Sophie Lycouris

The problematics

European Union has both direct and indirect implications for the development and promotion of dance in Europe. A close examination of the European Union's current position on arts and culture is relevant to issues of dance management in the European context. In this complex administrative environment, European dance faces a promising future; yet it is unavoidable that new problems emerge and the necessity to develop new practices and strategies becomes increasingly urgent.

The purpose of this chapter is to discuss the character of the new set of conditions for the development of dance in Europe. The term 'Europe' is employed in a historical and geographical sense rather than a political one defined by the borders of the European Union. The chapter sets out to argue that, within the current European context, 'dance' and 'Europe' are two dynamic entities in constant interaction. Within this perspective, the cultural and economic phenomenon of 'Dance in Europe' can be better described as an 'interface' between dance and Europe. This metaphor works well as it indicates the fluid and ever-changing character of this phenomenon. It refers to the fact that the development of dance in Europe does not only rely on effective dance (and/or other) policies; it also requires that dance professionals respond to the existing structures both sensibly and imaginatively. Dance in Europe is currently under development and its future depends equally upon the contribution of all the parties involved. With this assumption, it is easy to understand why an element of dialogue is necessary for the whole project to meet its aims fully. This chapter therefore sets out to contribute to this debate. By initiating, feeding, and participating in the dialogue between dance and Europe, it is one more way of making dance 'happen' in Europe.

By way of introduction, the discussion on dance development in Europe could be approached in three different ways:

1. To address the direct role and contribution of the European Union to the development of dance in member and non-member states within Europe. Questions that consider which actions are possible with the European Union structures and funding schemes, and how to approach funding more effectively, are likely to arise.

2. To examine the indirect role and contribution of the European Union to the development of dance in member and non-member states within Europe. The new political reality of 'Europe without frontiers' in the form of Single Market (introduced by the Single European Act in the mid-1980s and further consolidated with the Treaty of Maastricht, 1992) facilitates collaborations and exchanges between artists and companies in Europe.[1] A number of economic complications have disappeared as a result of the free circulation of money and people.

3. The final strand of debate encompasses experience of exchange between European countries. The idea of 'Europe without frontiers' offers a favourable environment for the consolidation and further development of linking mechanisms between European countries. In order to assist this objective, the Council of Europe has recently founded a European Resource Centre for Cultural Policies to complete a research project on the cultural policies of European countries, which was initiated in 1985.[2]

In order to understand the current state of affairs it is important to discuss the position of culture within the project of European integration prior to the Treaty of Maastricht.

Culture in Europe before the Maastricht Treaty

The fusion between cultural factors and other aspects of production is connected with the history of the European Union itself. Originally, the European Economic Community was an economic union. With the Single Market, goods were allowed to circulate freely among the member states. Cultural goods should normally follow the same rule; yet it soon became obvious that their free circulation would affect their national heritage (a crucial element of European culture) as these goods were permanently under risk of being removed from their 'native lands'. In the Netherlands, for example, selling paintings by Mondrian to collectors abroad could cause significant losses in the area of cultural heritage (Loman et al, 1992, p.24). For this reason, the European Community developed an appropriate legal framework for these member states, which set out 'to prevent the exportation of a work of art which they consider to be part of the national cultural heritage' (Loman et al, 1992, p.24). In practical terms, this solution was overtly against the aims of the free circulation of goods; there were many cases in which the Court of Justice had to make decisions within this contradictory domain simply based on their own sense of judgement (Loman et al, 1992, p.94).

While Europe was shifting from an economic union to a political one, it became increasingly evident that no clear distinction could be made between cultural and economic aspects of certain cultural products. In addition, there was a gradual recognition that the notion of culture was a crucial factor within the project of European integration (Loman et al, 1992). Initially, the populations of the different member states were resistant to this process because there were not enough links or common elements to bring them closer to each other and make them feel members of the same group. The notion of 'European identity' therefore became instrumental in this process. Initially, the common elements between the European nations were sought in the past, in history. Although theoretically Europeans belong to the same group, it is difficult to support this argument at the level of everyday experience. Europeans speak so many different languages and their most common shared experience is unfortunately the memory of fighting against each other during various wars. Consequently, there was no hope of constructing a 'European identity' by means of the past. An effort was then made to create it in the present using a number of simple devices: a European flag and shared activities, such as the European City of Culture and European Cultural Month.

In general, in the context of a united Europe, 'culture' was never treated as a distinct domain and action supporting culture was always consequential of action initiated in the context of other (primarily economic) policies. The Treaty of Maastricht introduced article 128, an article exclusively dedicated to cultural matters, which provided a clear rationale for the first European Cultural Policy.[3] Before looking at the implications of article 128 in more detail, the following section considers the impact of 'cultural policies' on dance.

The relationship between cultural policies and dance policies

A sound examination of national policies that currently support dance in Europe relies on an understanding of such notions as 'culture', 'art' and 'policy', and the relationships between cultural policies and dance policies. Loman et al (1992) introduces some of the fundamental issues as far as the term 'culture' is concerned. Traditionally 'culture' referred to 'the highest intellectual achievements of human beings' (Prott in Loman et al, 1992, p.2); more recently, anthropologists have redefined the term as:

> The totality of the knowledge and practices, both intellectual and material of each of the particular groups of a society and . . . itself as a whole.
>
> (Guillaumin in Loman et al, 1992, p.2)

According to this wider perspective, 'culture' refers to a vast range of human activities, one of which is artistic production.

The latter definition, however, has not yet motivated any radical revision of the term 'cultural policy',[4] which still primarily covers areas such as the development of the arts and possibly other intellectual activities.[5] At the present moment, there is no general consensus (or definition) on the term 'cultural policy'. Loman et al (1992, p.2) argue that, there is no need to 'embrace one specific definition [of cultural policy]'. They explain that the term refers to the totality of 'measures and actions which the Member States commonly take in pursuit of their objectives of cultural policy', relying on a number of different assumptions.[6]

Both in Europe and in other parts of the world, dance policies have often been considered as specific areas of broadly conceived cultural policies. In some cases, as for instance in the Greek Cultural Policy, guidelines for the development of dance are specifically included within cultural policy documents; yet they are often used only as examples that illustrate the potential implementation of the particular cultural policy. In these instances, although dance has been taken into account, there is no attention paid to dance's distinct features, in terms of its development, and therefore such references can not be considered as dance policies.

During the last 15 years, a number of European countries (including the UK and France) have put a special effort into identifying dance's specific needs in the areas of choreographic and audience development, distribution and access. This concern has resulted in the birth of strategies conceived exclusively in order to support the development of dance; these can be considered as typical examples of dance policy. In other cases, dance policy is non-existent and any development of dance is the result of a number of 'personal' interpretations and implementations of a generic cultural policy. This situation has some advantages, in the sense that it is open to creative solutions. Yet, because it is beyond the scope of such generic policies to suggest specific developmental models for individual art forms, they cannot support dance's development in any specific ways. They provide no clarity about what should be done or what could be achieved in the area of dance development, and it remains a matter of the user's personal skill to find effective ways to apply the general guidelines in order to address the development of dance. In these cases, dance shares the 'funding pie' with a wide range of other cultural activities and frequently fails to gain funding.

This is because other domains, such as theatre, music and film, are often prioritised on the basis that they appeal to larger numbers of people. The main task of anyone interested in the development of dance is then to convince both state and private sponsors that dance is also part of the cultural scene.

In European countries, generic cultural policies (that fail to offer suggestions about the development of individual art forms) are no longer popular and tend to have been replaced by area specific policies that pursue area-specific objectives at national level.[7] At European level, however, the generic cultural policy model has been recognised as the most effective in supporting the arts nationally, regionally and locally, without interfering too much with the complex and diverse cultural landscape of Europe. This means that there can be no dance policy at European Union level as there can be no other area-specific arts policy. Consequently, dance can only benefit from the European Union's general emphasis on culture and, in practical terms, this means that again dance has to share the 'funding pie' with other areas of cultural activity, including tourism.[8] Yet in the context of European Union, as with other art forms, dance can also benefit from funds originally designed to fulfil completely different purposes. This is probably a unique feature of the European Union and brings to the surface some unusual strategies for promoting dance, including action undertaken not only outside any notion of dance policy, but even beyond any sense of cultural policy as well.[9]

European Cultural Policy and the Treaty of Maastricht: the emphasis on culture

Article 128 of the Maastricht treaty, which focuses exclusively on cultural matters, includes five paragraphs in which a double concern becomes evident: on the one hand, the European Union recognises the need to support national cultures, but on the other, the need to promote the notion of 'European identity' and a common 'European culture'. Article 128 clearly states this double aim and emphasises the importance of collaboration between the member states so that, according to the principle of subsidiality,[10] the European Union does not have to interfere in the internal problems of member states.

In article 128, it is also mentioned that the European Union can support the 'artefacts' of European Culture or common heritage, books and audio-visual production. The principle of subsidiarily is further emphasised by pointing out that no harmonisation[11] of the national cultural policies should take place; the European Union pursues cultural policy objectives by means of advice and recommendation. The notion of cultural co-operation is also introduced and it is explicitly stated that an important aspect of the European Union's cultural policy is to collaborate on cultural matters at both European and international level. Yet the most important element of the article, which is essentially of theoretical and philosophical importance, is the idea that the cultural factor should be taken into consideration in the making of any other policy in the Union.[12] This obviously has implications for the development of dance in Europe.

The European Union's funding of culture

On the basis of the principles introduced in article 128, the European Union identified three areas of priority in pursuing its cultural policy cultural heritage; books and reading; and artistic activities (including the performing arts). From a dance perspective, this situation does not seem promising at first glance, as it does not take into account the specific problems and conditions of supporting dance in Europe and does not suggest any area-specific development models for individual art forms. Yet the generic nature of the article, in combination with the principle of subsidiarity,[13] clearly introduces the European Union's role in the development of the arts in Europe as a supportive one; it provides a loose framework within which there is plenty of space for national cultural policies to meet their context-specific responsibilities and for area-specific initiatives to emerge and flourish.

A number of such initiatives have taken place in the domain of dance in the form of exchange programmes, common platforms, co-productions or forums. The Informal European Theatre Meeting (IETM) has become one of the most important forums for the development of dance at European level. At least once a year, it brings together a large number of dance artists, as well as producers and promoters. In this way, it provides one of the most recognised 'informal' contexts in which European dance is promoted in Europe. IETM, comprising more than 300 theatre and dance organisations from 40 different countries, has become the main channel through which a vast number of imaginative solutions for the promotion of dance have emerged. One of the areas in which IETM demonstrates some interesting work is a list of basic points outlining how the development of theatre and dance in Europe should be pursued. This material has become part of the document *Theatre and Dance in the 1990s* published by IETM (1992) and can play the role of a suggestive generic policy for the development of theatre and dance in Europe, in the sense that it has no legal character, nor does it refer to specific projects that are expected to achieve this purpose. Some of the most important points are as follows:

- It is important to establish communication networks, to be in touch with the most recent information, to learn from other people's experiences, and to establish inter-governmental agencies that will support cross-border initiatives. Local authorities should be encouraged to support local production.
- The participation of dance professionals who have been largely excluded from the process of the decisions should be encouraged. The European Union is a large organisation operating within rigid bureaucratic structures. Often crucial information, which determines the character of the formal decision about distribution of funds, is repeatedly processed through a series of administrative steps, therefore losing the clarity of the original points and the direct contact with the professional or other groups involved.
- Exchange of knowledge, information and experience should be developed in order to facilitate the process of applying for European money in the arts. In addition, mobility should be encouraged through supporting touring projects and other opportunities of exchanging expertise, such as workshops, meetings, etc.
- A model for theatre and dance development should be constructed. This is not (and should not be) the European Union's responsibility, and therefore the professionals should themselves undertake the task, with long-term financial support provided by the European Union.

With this last point, the IETM seems to accept the fact that European Cultural Policy, as articulated in the Maastricht Treaty, cannot (and should not) do anything beyond the provision of a suggestive and supportive framework for the development of the arts in Europe. Yet in another document, *Bread and Circuses: EC programmes open to the performing arts*, also published by IETM (1992), a number of suggestions have been made, to facilitate the work of a prospective European funding seeker for the support of the arts, in a tone that implies the organisation's discontent with the current situation. Some of these suggestions emphasise the importance of lobbying and being in direct contact with officers in Brussels (where all the main decisions on the distribution of funds are usually taken) as well as the necessity of knowing 'how to read between the lines'. It is true that these skills are crucial in seeking funding for the arts from the European Union and this can sometimes create the wrong impression, suggesting that the procedures according to which the distribution of funds takes place within the European Union are not fair or taken seriously enough.

It is important to remember though that lobbying, networking and, to some extent, guessing, risking and betting on what might be the true agenda behind any application guidelines are standard practices of fund-raising methods. Moreover, concepts, policies and (therefore funds) at European Union level are much more generic in character as their aim is to stimulate creative implementation and allow for national, regional and local differences to be taken into account. This is why they are more open to interpretation and imaginative applications, which is not necessarily a bad thing. In particular, the fact that a large number of non-culture-based European funds can be (and have been) used in arts projects again demonstrates the generic character of these funds, as well as the broadness and imagination with which their guidelines can be interpreted. This peculiarity of the European Union funding system acknowledges both theoretically and practically the artists' constant desire that art should not be an isolated activity in current society; on the contrary, it should be treated seriously and on equal terms with other traditionally more important aspects of everyday life and as a crucial part of the social domain. The Appendix at the end of this chapter lists some of the non-culture based funds that could be applied to dance at present.[14]

There is, however, one European Union funding scheme created exclusively for the support of the arts in Europe that can be used (and has been used) for the support of dance projects: KALEIDOSCOPE.[15] There has been much discussion recently in relation to the effectiveness of the programme and a number of changes have been suggested. At present its objectives are as follows:

- to encourage activities involving artistic creation with a European dimension;
- to support innovative cultural projects carried out by European partners from at least three different member states;
- to contribute to the development of the professional skills of artists and other cultural operators; and
- to contribute to mutual knowledge of European cultures.

(Official Journal of the European Communities, 1996, p.17).

It is interesting to note that dance-based projects are increasingly supported by KALEIDOSCOPE. In 1997, Lloyd Newson's British dance company, DV8 Physical Theatre, became one of the most important recipients of the KALEIDOSCOPE scheme for a dance-based project that brought together five European partners under the initiative of the company's managing director, Leonie Gombrich (1997). Gombrich (1997) is convinced that, for these applications to be successful, the applicant needs to be really fresh and imaginative, and to be able to put together a project specifically conceived for KALEIDOSCOPE's criteria: 'I read about the KALEIDOSCOPE and even the way their guidelines were worded gave me some ideas.' In DV8's case, the application was made around the idea of technology and communication. During the early choreographic stages of *Bound to Please* (1997):

> There was a lot [of talk] about breaking the fourth wall, making the audience unsure about was what happening on stage as part of the show and what was part of the real experience . . . a lot about whether technology distances people or brings them closer together.
>
> Gombrich (1997)

Not all of these ideas ultimately survived in the piece, but this starting point was sufficient to stimulate Gombrich's thinking towards the idea of a website; this included some live sessions, during which the choreographer Lloyd Newson could receive messages and questions through the Internet and respond to them. In the end, the majority of the KALEIDOSCOPE money was spent on making and running the website, but other portions of it were used to enhance the show technologically with additional elements, such as projections, that would not have happened otherwise. Another area which benefited from the same fund was the promotion of the work. Many different and imaginative ideas were used around Europe to promote DV8's work to audiences such as students and other young people. *Bound to Please* was a genuine 'European' production, as is most of DV8's work: it was co-produced by five producers from London, Cambridge, Utrecht, Paris and Angers, all of whom participated in the KALEIDOSCOPE application.

John Ashford (1997), artistic director of *Resolution!* at The Place Theatre in London, has also applied twice to KALEIDOSCOPE, but without success. He agrees with Gombrich that the most important point in getting KALEIDOSCOPE support is to submit projects that have been exclusively made to fit the criteria; yet according to him this is a very narrow-minded approach. *Aerowaves*,[16] which is part of the *Resolution!* programme, was never specifically conceived to fit the KALEIDOSCOPE criteria. Instead, it was an idea born from specific needs in the area of promoting young choreographers in Europe. Ashford believes that this was the reason why his applications were unsuccessful and sees this as problematic. His idea of *Aerowaves* had a very sound basis as far as the European element was concerned; yet he believes that it was ultimately considered 'on geo-political grounds', rather than artistic ones, which have often banned big European cities from operating as leaders of KALEIDOSCOPE projects.[17]

A comparison between DV8's production *Bound to Please* and the *Aerowaves* project, in tenor of their success and failure with the KALEIDO-SCOPE scheme, is interesting; not only because it brings to the fore a number of positive and negative points in relation to European funds for the arts, but it also puts into context a number of burning issues as far as the current situation of the development of dance in Europe is concerned.

Within a KALEIDOSCOPE application, the selection of European partners (which should total at least three) is a key point. John Ashford believes that 'geo-political reasons' keep major European cities excluded from the fund, but this cannot explain why DV8, a London-based company, was successful with the application. It seems more plausible, therefore, that the main reason for *Aerowaves'* failure was that the project had not been exclusively conceived in order to fulfil the KALEIDOSCOPE criteria. At first glance, this seems a narrow-minded framework; yet it is important to remember that an important objective of European Cultural Policy is to strengthen 'European Identity' through supporting European arts, rather than supporting the arts in a general way. This means that the European Union expects a number of projects to be specifically designed to fulfil this purpose. Although for some people like John Ashford this might be a sterile exercise, for others like Leonie Gombrich the same restriction becomes an interesting stimulus. There is, however, a lot of grey area around this discussion in the sense that, from the perspective of the European Union, there is an implied assumption that by fulfilling the KALEIDOSCOPE's highly debated criteria automatically means that the successful projects support the notion of 'European Identity'.

In the above comparison, there is no reason why *Aerowaves* could not be considered as a good means to support this European integration project, in a way that is very different from the DV8 project, but is equally significant. Moreover, it seems plausible that if the DV8 co-production was successful with KALEIDOSCOPE because it encouraged cultural exchange and established lasting co-operation among the five partners involved (two crucial elements in the selection process), there is no good explanation as to why *Aerowaves* did not fulfil the same criteria. In fact, *Aerowaves* brought together a much larger group of Europeans, not only during the preparation phase (22 partners), but also in the outcome: a large number of dancers and choreographers from all over Europe had the opportunity to meet, exchange experiences, and to establish professional and social relationships for future collaborations.

Another issue that is highlighted by the above discussion is the connection between the direct economic and political implications of the European integration project led by the European Union itself and the development of a European spirit which features in various aspects of current life, including artistic production. John Ashford emphasises the role of English language, which has become increasingly dominant in the European context, facilitating communications in this way. He also notes that cheap air flights within the area of Europe have significantly encouraged travelling and therefore create favourable conditions for contact, exchange and general mobility; this has brought Europeans closer together and helped them become part of the same group. Ashford is not convinced by the argument that the European Union procedures, and the political and financial conditions that it has established in Europe, should be indebted for this positive situation. Yet Leonie Gombrich enthuses over the advantages of working at European level.

The first aspect of this experience is the opportunity for multiple funding and the chance to reach multinational audiences, which offers greater potential for a piece of work to become successful. European co-productions also offer her the chance to work closely with other European promoters, dance managers and organisers, therefore enriching her own skills with a wide range of new and inspirational working methods. At this point, it is important to mention that DV8's connection with European producers and audiences is not new and is not only an outcome of the company's recent success with the KALEIDOSCOPE application. Yet, the fact that the company has managed to work in Europe with such consistency in the course of its 11-year-old life is very much a direct consequence of the Single Market, initiated by the European Community in the 1980s and consolidated by the European Union in the early 1990s.

Several lessons can be drawn from the study of two essentially European projects, despite their failure or success with the KALEIDO-SCOPE programme. Firstly, there is potential for a wide range of interpretations of what a 'European' project might be, and which techniques should be followed for such projects to be successfully funded by European sources. Secondly, the European Union administrative structures need to become increasingly open and supportive to work produced by dance professionals within Europe, which often acquires a strong European character without being necessarily conceived in order to fulfil a European fund's criteria.

British dance in the wider Europe

In this new landscape of dance development in Europe, the position of British dance acquires a new significance. On the one hand, British dance faces a number of threats or even challenges, because of the high level of competition. On the other hand, it becomes obvious that British dance has unique elements to contribute to, and shape, this phenomenon of 'dance in Europe'. Rod Fisher (1992c) has identified some of the key points in this area.

Mobility

Fisher (1992c) argues that free mobility of performers should stimulate employment and improve the position of the artist. Although in practice, foreign companies are expensive by British standards, the opposite might happen. Good quality companies with low rates and can threaten the selling power of British dance within the UK. At the same time, the opposite is true as far as technical staff are concerned: there is a serious problem of technical staff leaving Britain because salaries in this field are much higher abroad. Fisher (1992c) also questions how the frequent presence of foreign companies in Britain might affect audience expectations in terms of the kind of work they expect to see from British companies. This forms another kind of competition.

Funding

Fisher (1992c) suggests that British dance companies do not get enough financial support to be able to cope with touring abroad whereas other countries, such as France, have established special measures to achieve maximum exportation. From this perspective, British dance is again in a weak position. Likewise, British promoters cannot afford to travel in Europe to identify interesting companies for their programmes; and even if they could, British venues could not afford the high fees of good quality Continental dance. In addition, there have been cases in which the Inland Revenue was not consistent in dealing with taxation of income from touring abroad and the VAT issue is still largely unresolved.

Currently Britain is trying to adapt to this new set of conditions by introducing radical changes. Initially Britain created a Department of National Heritage in order to comply with similar structures of member states of the European Union, which in 1997 became the Department of Culture, Media and Sports. Secondly, the British Council has launched a policy on international arts. Fisher (1992c) contends that, because this was done under pressure, the policy is not concrete.

In this highly competitive landscape, one way of promoting British dance in Europe would be to highlight areas in which Britain is experienced and has been successful. There are a number of important areas that could be used towards this aim, such as non-Western dance, community dance practice, and integrated dance work between able-bodied and disabled performers. In 1991, the British Council, in collaboration with the Arts Council and the European Community, offered 'Black' travel grants to promote Black Arts in Europe. In addition the debate around the development of British dance has much to offer the development of dance in Europe. British dance policy can demonstrate unique strategies in the support of new and experimental dance, through specifically designed training programmes and institutions such as the National Dance Agencies (NDAs).

Diversity

A crucial topic, in which British dance experts are again more experienced than their European colleagues, is the critique of the dominance of Western dance forms (such as ballet) in the British context (Fisher, 1992c). The strong presence of South Asian and African Peoples' dance in the UK has inevitably made visible the cultural basis of Western dance and thus revealed the myth that ballet is a 'universal' art form. At the same time, as South Asian and African Peoples' dance occupy a considerable part of British dance, this has offered the British dance audience an opportunity to become familiar with them and, consequently, learn how to appreciate their artistic value. In the European context this discussion becomes a critique of Eurocentricism.

Fisher (1992c) notes that Eurocentricism threatens minority cultures in Europe and undermines commonalities with other cultures outside Europe (such as New Zealand and other Commonwealth countries). Europe seems to be in permanent risk of becoming a 'Fortress Europe' and gradually eliminating cultural exchange with non-EU countries. Choreographer Shobana Jeyasingh (in Arts Council et al, 1990, vol. 6) believes that minority arts should not be supported as a matter of obligation, but because of their artistic value. This means they should be considered as part of the whole European picture, which is not the case at all in the current situation. In this respect, Fisher (1992c) suggests that European cultural policy should not aim at a diversity of European cultures, but at a diversity of cultures in Europe.

Conclusion

The purpose of this chapter was to introduce the complex character of the discussion about the development of dance in the current European context, given the political and economic changes that have been introduced with European Union in a post-Maastricht era. It has been suggested that this debate relates to (at least) two elements: firstly, it covers the close examination of the effect of the European Union structures on the development of dance through the introduction of new political and economic conditions, the development of a basic European Cultural Policy, and the availability of a number of funding schemes; secondly, it encompasses the potential for exchange, communication and co-operation, supported by the free circulation of people, money, products and services in the area of Europe.

European Union structures provide only indirect support for the development of dance, as there is no dedicated dance (or any other area-specific) arts policy at European level. This is primarily because the main purpose of European Cultural Policy is to provide a supportive framework within which implementation can take place according to the specificity of national, regional and local parameters. This condition has created a peculiarly loose situation in relation to the development of the arts (and therefore dance) in Europe, which often gives the impression that there is very little that can be achieved. Through detailed reference to two European dance-based British projects, this chapter argues that there is much room for interpretation and creative work, as well as for improvement both in relation to the use of European funds and the understanding of what is (or could be) the character of European dance. There is a lot to be done in this area; European dance has not found an identity yet and cannot be defined simply by means of funding structures and available supportive policies.

To a large extent, the development of dance in Europe is a matter of understanding the complexity, as well as the potential, of the current situation and developing fresh and imaginative working methods that will be able to meet this challenge. In this process, there is much to be learnt through experiencing exchange at the level of different models of supporting dance in Europe, and Britain's contribution in this area can be seminal.

Notes

1. There are alternative opinions about this phenomenon. For instance, John Ashford (1997) argues that the main reason why exchange between artists and companies has become increasingly easier is not 'Europe without frontiers', but mainly cheap air travel and the dominance of English language.
2. This chapter does not include this kind of comparative study, as it would have been impossible to give sufficient attention to this past of the discussion within its limits. A comparative analysis between the French and British dance policies has been introduced in my paper *Comparing Dance Policies: British and French Approaches* (1997b).
3. For further details about the position of culture in pre-Maastricht Europe in relation to its history and structures, please see another version of this chapter entitled *Dance in Europe* (1997a). Research papers on Dance Policy and Management, Department of Dance Studies, University of Surrey.
4. If this has already happened in some cases it remains, nevertheless, an exception.
5. For example, the Maastricht Treaty has introduced a number of areas which the European Cultural Policy should support, including books and reading.
6. The fact that European Cultural Policy operates according to the principle of *subsidiarity* explains why this inclusive attitude is both necessary and

unproblematic. See note 10 for further explanation on subsidiarity.

7. An exception to this rule is the current situation in Germany where there is clearly no interest in dealing with dance policy at national level. Dance development has become a purely regional issue and this is why a number of different models are regionally applied towards this aim.

8. At first glance it seems quite peculiar that there have been cases in which the development of tourism has been used as a rationale for supporting dance. Yet one can at least partially explain this peculiarity under the light of the redefinition of the term 'culture' (as explained earlier in the paper), which has established a broader notion of 'culture' including a range of both intellectual and material aspects of productive activities.

9. For examples of cultural projects (of which very few are dance-based) please see the directory *More Bread and Circuses* published by ETM (1994).

10. Subsidiarity is the principle according to which a 'decision should be taken at the lowest possible appropriate level – that is at local, regional and national, rather than E[uropean]C[ommunity] level' (ETM, 1991, p. 100). This means that national policies should primarily provide the main guidelines for action in all areas except those in which only a common strategy at European level could be really effective, as is environmental policy for example.

11. In harmonisation, all variations of national laws dealing with a specific domain need to conform to the European law because this is the only way to provide quick and safe solutions. Because of the principle of subsidiarity, however, harmonisation is applied as little as possible and in those cases in which it seems absolutely necessary, such as Environmental Policy.

12. This is an important point because it can justify why funding for other purposes could be also used for cultural purposes.

13. See notes 6 and 10.

14. European funding programmes and schemes change from year to year, sometimes quite radically. This means that it is absolutely imperative for the individuals or organisations who wish to apply have access to the most recent information. Directories of funding schemes such as *Bread and Circuses* or *Sources of European Community Funding* are not safe sources unless their most recent editions are available. An alternative solution is to consult the monthly directories of the European Union which lists new publications and documents. These documents can be found in the Official Journal and they include all the necessary information, as well as samples of the application forms. The difficulty is to identify these documents and understand their relevance to culture, but this is an area one can improve only through experience. This kind of information is usually kept in the Documentation Centres of the European Union, the addresses of which can be found in central offices of the European Union, such as the London Office.

15. The KALEIDOSCOPE scheme replaced PLATFORM EUROPE, an earlier European funding scheme with similar aims.

16. 'Aerowaves was set up in response to the burgeoning expansion of contemporary dance being made by young choreographers and companies across Europe. Its original aim was to offer an opportunity for those emerging artists to tour

outside their country and gain experience by presenting their work in a different cultural context' (*Aerowaves* 1996/7 Report). *Aerowaves* has been managed, originally, by a group of 22 partners (they then became 28) from all over Europe under the leadership and initiative of John Ashford. In 1996, when this festival was launched, 150 applicants from all over Europe submitted work and, from those, ten were finally selected through a carefully planned procedure. The feedback was very positive after this first attempt; yet this did not seem to affect the decisions at European Union level and the project was rejected one more time, despite the relatively small amount that has been asked: from £13000 of total cost, the amount of £8000 had been requested from the KALEIDOSCOPE programme.

17. A large number of European funding schemes in various areas (and not exclusively in the arts) prioritise disadvantaged and poor European regions, such as South Europe or heavily industrial and proletarian urban areas, such as the towns of Leeds and Liverpool in the UK, in order to give them more chances to improve the quality of life of the populations living in these areas. In this sense, in a KALEIDOSCOPE application, it is important to include a number of partners from such areas in order to give them a fair chance to learn from the experience of the others.

Appendix

Non-culture based funds that could be applied to dance

- SOCIAL FUND: this fund is not directly available to individuals, but rather to local authorities, government departments or voluntary sectors, from which individuals should ask information and to which they should submit applications.

- LEI (Local Employment Initiative for Women): this fund supports women through financial awards and other employment-creation initiatives, in setting up their own businesses.

- ERASMUS: this fund is aimed at promoting the European dimension in universities and encouraging mobility of students.

- LEONARDO DA VINCI: this programme aims to support quality and innovation in Member states vocational training systems through transnational training partnerships between training bodies and firms, and transnational placement and exchange programmes.

- MEDIA: this programme is designed to stimulate a European audiovisual industry. Through its 19 schemes, it supports the training of European professionals, the development, promotion, distribution and exhibition of European productions, the restoration and use of European archive and the development of new technology.

- TIDE: The aim is to develop and validate systems and services allowing the integration of elderly and disabled people. The project supports research, development and demonstration projects and the use of advanced information and communication technologies including robotics, mobility control systems, prosthetics and orthotics devices to increase the autonomy and improve the quality of life of disabled and elderly people.

European Commission (UK) 1995

References

Arts Council of England et al (1990) *Arts without frontiers: effects on the arts of the European Single Market*, Conference Proceedings, Glasgow: Arts Council of England, *Sunday Times* and British Council, March (vols 1, 2, 5, 6, 7, 9, 10, 12, 17, 19, 20).

Ashford, J. (1997) Interview with Sophie Lycouris on Aerowaves project (part of *Resolution* dance festival), London, The Place Theatre, 29 August.

Bainbridge, T. and Teasdale, A. (1995) *The Penguin Companion to European Union*, London: Penguin.

Fisher, R. (1992a) *Who does what in Europe?*, London: The Arts Council of England.

—— (1992b) *Arts networking in Europe*, London: The Arts Council of England.

—— (1992c) *Challenge for the arts: reflections on British Culture in Europe in the context of the Single Market & Maastricht*, London: Arts Council of England.

Gombrich, L. (1997) Interview with Sophie Lycouris on DV8's application to KALEIDOSCOPE funding scheme, London, Toynbee Studios, 1 September.

IETM (1991) *Theatre and dance in the 1990s*, Brussels: Informal European Theatre Meeting (IETM).

—— (1992) *Bread and Circuses: EC programmes and schemes open to the performing arts*, Brussels: IETM.

—— (1994) *More Bread and Circuses: who does what for the arts in Europe*, London: Arts Council of England/IETM.

Loman, J. et al (1992) *Culture and Community law: before and after Maastricht*, Deventer & Boston: Kluwer Law and Taxation Publishers.

Lycouris, S. (1997a) 'Dance in Europe', in *Research Papers on Dance Policy and Management*, no. 4, University of Surrey: Department of Dance Studies.

—— (1997b) 'Comparing Dance Policies: British and French Approaches', *Research Papers on Dance Policy and Management*, no. 5, University of Surrey: Department of Dance Studies.

—— (1996) Official Journal of the European Communities, *European Community support for culture – 1996 Kaleidoscope programme – Information and call for applications*, OJ C114, vol. 39, 19 April, pp.16–20.

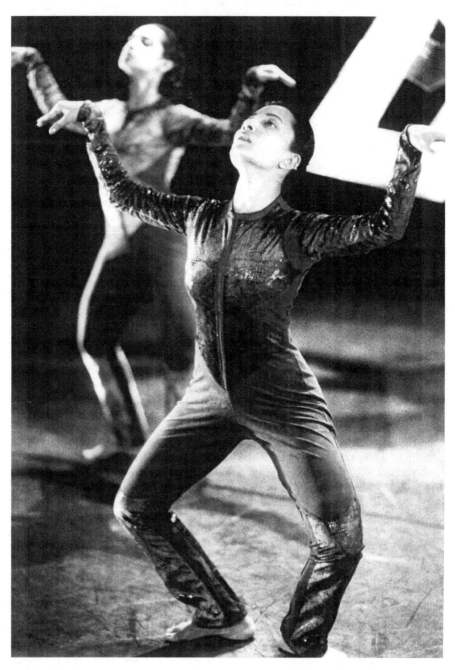

Shobana Jeyasingh Dance Company

13

Made in Britain: Home and Away

Sue Hoyle

This chapter is a personal perspective on strategies for developing the profile of British dance in Europe, which draws on my experience of working in Paris for a year. My time there suggested there was a need to increase the promotion of British dance in France, as there may be in other European countries, and to offer further opportunities for exchange between choreographers, dancers and programmers.

Very few British choreographers are known in France. Those who are, tend to give one-off performances in provincial festivals; only a handful are invited to perform in Paris. At the capital's 'dance house', the Théâtre de la Ville, the work of French choreographers is seen alongside that of companies from many countries, and DV8 was recently invited to appear there, but, by and large, invitations to other British companies are extremely rare. Nor is this apparent lack of interest in Britain's dance confined to contemporary choreographers or small, lesser-known groups. Large dance companies from around the world perform at venues in the capital: for example, Merce Cunningham at the Palais Garnier and Frankfurt Ballet at the Châtelet, but it has been many years since any of Britain's mainstream dance companies performed in Paris.

What is the reason for such poor representation of British dance in France? There may be several explanations:

- Different methods of public funding in the two countries
- Cultural and aesthetic differences
- Inadequate promotion and publicity.

These factors will now be considered in more detail.

Funding

In Britain, we tend to assume that dance in France is well funded, with grants focused on creation and with little pressure to tour extensively. But that is only part of the story. The way in which public funding for dance creation is organised in France and Britain differs. In France there is much greater investment in culture by the state than there is in Britain, and many choreographers and dancers benefit from substantial funds available at local and regional level, as well as those given through the Ministry of Culture and other government departments. There is little business sponsorship for the arts in France, and only minimal reliance on earned income. There was a move to decentralise funding in the 1980s and a confidence-boosting celebration of the art form in *L'Année de la Danse* in 1988. Artist-led choreographic centres were established. In Britain, the dance economy is far more mixed. A recent survey by the Arts Council of England of 42 regularly funded dance companies shows that they earned 37 per cent of their total income, mainly through performance fees and ticket sales; 10 per cent was 'contributed' (usually through sponsorship); and only 5 per cent overall came from local authorities. Unlike France, British dance has access to lottery funds made available nationally through schemes such as the *Arts for Everyone* programme. As regards the distribution of government grants, the categories of funding offered by the Arts Council of England reflect the relationship between the funded and the funder. Although there are a few one-off grants in areas such as training, 'black dance' development and youth arts, the main groupings are national, regularly funded, fixed-term funded and, very broadly, independent projects.

Funding by the French Ministry of Culture appears, from the outside at least, to be directed more strategically towards particular ends. The Ministry recently published an analysis of some 80 million French francs spent on choreographer-led companies in 1996. Seventeen national choreographic centres received between them about 54 million francs, but although the focus of their work was dance creation, they were expected to demonstrate a commitment to training and developing the public's interest in their work. Just under ten million francs was directed towards artistic research and development, with 26 established companies receiving modest funds for two years, but having no obligation to make a new dance work every year. The funds for the 80 companies receiving project grants (30 of them for the first time) were directed primarily towards creation, without the same demands for performance as we find in Britain. The average grant, however, was much lower (the equivalent of about £8000 in France compared to £24000 in Britain). Other funding programmes were directed towards repertory development for ballet companies based in regional opera houses. Choreographic residencies were supported: some were linked to audience development and others were associated with arts organisations with a producing and touring role, such as the Maison de la Culture in Amiens and the Merlan Theatre in Marseilles.

Culture

It is assumed that one of the reasons for such poor representation in France by British dance companies is that French promoters and producers have different artistic tastes from British ones. Indeed, historically, here are many differences between Britain and France in terms of aesthetics, infrastructure and operation, it is easy to assume that this may be the case. In Britain, the influence of choreographers and teachers such as Ashton, Graham and Cunningham is evident in many dance companies, as are dance forms from the Caribbean, South Asia and Africa, whereas in France Béjart, Nikolais, and Bausch & Hip Hop would be equivalent influences.

Although relatively well-supported through public funding, dance in France has little focus in formal education; it is much less well-established in secondary and higher education than it is in Britain. Young people, however, are developing a strong dance culture, particularly within the Arab/North African and Latin American communities, living on the outskirts of big cities. Many young people's dances are inspired by hip-hop and some groups have already received funding from the French government.

In France, there is less of a divide between mainstream ballet and contemporary dance than there is in Britain. Indeed, established contemporary choreographers are probably considered to make up the mainstream whereas in Britain they are often described as 'independent'. Contemporary choreographers such as Maguy Marin, Angelin Preljocaj and Jean-Claude Gallotta create work for classical ballet companies where their work reaches large audiences and is seen alongside international peers such as Bill T. Jones, Stephen Petronio or Susan Marshall. No contemporary British choreographer is in evidence in the French ballet repertory.

As in Britain, dance is pioneering participation in the arts ahead of many other disciplines, and dance from the 'banlieues' is leading in this area. For example, in spring 1996, the Parc de la Villette, in the north of Paris, organised a festival called 'Rencontres Nationales de Danse Urbaines'. It featured dance groups formed by young people from many French cities. The programme was created by and for young people. This festival was so successful that the next 'Rencontres' (in autumn 1997) was extended to include general urban culture as well as dance. Theatre, writing, visual arts, outdoor performance and video were added, although dance continued to outstrip the other forms in terms of attendances. Future festivals will have more of an international dimension and should provide an opportunity for British youth dance groups to be involved.

Funding programmes in France indicate that the French government seems to have an interest in public access as well as creativity. A 1996 survey on dance by the Association Française D'Action Artistique stated that many established choreographers wanted to tour more, their work was dealing increasingly with social issues, and they were starting to choreograph for different settings, such as prisons. In March 1998, the Minister of Culture issued a consultative document on funding of the performing arts, which placed great emphasis on access through education, training and enablement.

While French ballet companies attract reasonable audiences for new work, contemporary companies do not always attract a large public. Indeed, outside Paris, most companies perform for one night only, unless they are appearing in festivals or at the Maison de la Danse in Lyon. Such opportunities are few and far between for British companies, most of whom therefore perform in French cities for one performance at a time, which is clearly disadvantageous in terms of economics and profile-raising.

How does this snapshot of dance in France compare to our perception of the current state of dance in Britain? We are proud of our diversity and track record in community dance, but British choreographers seem to lack the confidence and self-esteem of their French counterparts. Working conditions are poor, funding seems inadequate and the divide between established companies (particularly classical ballet) and the rest of dance appears enormous. The move in the 1990s to develop a regional infrastructure though the establishment of National Dance Agencies (NDAs) is very different from the French model. In the main, NDAs are not led by choreographers, but by professionals with a background in dance programming, education or community dance. There are limited opportunities in Britain to experience live dance from overseas, and visiting companies are not normally integrated within a regular dance programme in the way they are, for instance, at the Théâtre de la Ville. Instead they tend to be presented within special seasons or festivals.

Raising the profile of British dance abroad

It may be true to say that French programmers are not aware of the diversity and originality of current British dance. If they do not have the opportunity to experience British dance, and are not in touch with dance programmers in Britain, they will remain unaware of the opportunities British dance has to offer, especially if they are not reached effectively by the promotional and marketing efforts of our dance companies.

Researchers who recently conducted an export market analysis for the British Council found that Britain was regarded as traditional, backward-looking and conventional. The British Council claims the arts are excellent ambassadors, and that dance itself is able to break down language barriers and refresh current international perceptions of Britain. Dance today can help position Britain in Europe as a vital, dynamic, culturally diverse and up-to-date nation. A recent article in *The Independent* highlighted some of the key positive messages we should communicate about contemporary Britain. It suggested, for instance, that we are a creative island, combining a history of eccentricity with an ethos that values individuality, non-conformity and new ideas; we are a hybrid nation, thriving on diversity and using it to renew and refresh ourselves; and we can think big and be brave. We are global pacesetters in design, fashion and music, therefore why not dance?

Current British dance is well placed to promote the first and second of these points (creative originality and diversity) and, with increased self-esteem and targeted investment, we might go some way to feeling more courageous and 'thinking big'. We should not forget that, across the world, demand for live performance from Britain exceeds our ability to supply it. This is due partly to the limited availability of many British performing groups. British funders could re-examine the purpose of funding and consider the relative importance of reaching the taxpayers in the UK through extensive touring (sometimes to inappropriate venues, where audiences are not yet ready to see the work). Instead, funders could do more to promote British arts to audiences overseas.

The difference of emphasis between dance in France and Britain can be used to an advantage. In the past we spoke of foreign touring, taking our art to a different public, promoting Britain overseas. Now we speak of cultural exports, but the approach is the same, even if the language differs.

Conclusion

British dance companies have an uphill struggle trying to secure bookings in countries such as France. Improved marketing and increased awareness will help, but there are other ways of integrating British dance into the European 'marketplace'. Models in other art forms show the value of artistic collaboration, with artists from different countries creating work together that appeals to audiences across Europe, as well as enabling artists to spark creatively from one another. This kind of project is already familiar to opera producers and is becoming more frequent in theatre.

Dance is about people, not products, and is in a good position to promote 'people to people' diplomacy in efforts focused on creative collaboration, dialogue and exchange. In order for this to happen, some changes of attitude and funding structure need to happen. We must decide whether we have the appropriate networks and infrastructure. Are we willing to think bigger than British, to be mobile, flexible, communicate in other languages and plan in the longer term about new ways of working together?

The capacity for British dance to realise its full potential in France depends on a number of factors. These include:

- investment in production and export;
- identifying our strengths and promoting our unique characteristics;
- an understanding of overseas markets and the local dance infrastructure;
- plugging into networks of European promoters and understanding their interests and objectives; and
- flexibility and a willingness to collaborate.

It is up to those of us who have key roles as managers, administrators and promoters of dance, to communicate and demonstrate our commitment to these ideals, and thus to ensure a positive future for dance in Britain.

Index

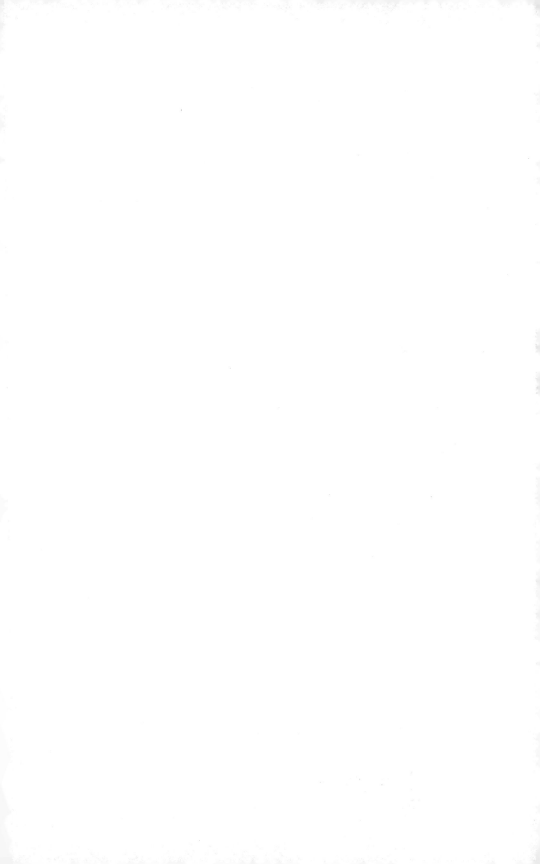

Lightning Source UK Ltd.
Milton Keynes UK
UKOW04f0004140614

233367UK00001B/52/P